Living with HIV

Living with HIV

A Patient's Guide

MARK CICHOCKI, RN

McFarland & Company, Inc., Publishers
Jefferson, North Carolina, and London

LIBRARY OF CONGRESS CATALOGUING-IN-PUBLICATION DATA

Cichocki, Mark, 1961–
    Living with HIV : a patient's guide / Mark Cichocki, RN.
      p.   cm.
    Includes bibliographical references and index.

    ISBN 978-0-7864-3921-8
    softcover : 50# alkaline paper ∞

    1. HIV-positive persons.   2. AIDS (Disease) — Patients.
3. Self-care, Health.   I. Title.
RA643.8.C53   2009
616.97'92 — dc22   2009008041

British Library cataloguing data are available

Cover photographs ©2009 Shutterstock

Manufactured in the United States of America

*McFarland & Company, Inc., Publishers
  Box 611, Jefferson, North Carolina 28640
  www.mcfarlandpub.com*

To my wife Bobbi and children
Amanda, Ashely, Lindsay, and Brandon.
They supported me in my efforts, showed confidence
in my abilities, and provided love throughout the process.

Contents

Introduction — Why Is This Book Needed?

Judith Rabkin, PhD., author of the book *Good Patients, Good Doctors*, summed it up in one sentence: "The patient's first major task after learning he or she is HIV positive is self-education."

Self-education not only enables people to go on with their lives, but allows them to make informed decisions regarding their own HIV care and empowers them, making them critical members of the healthcare team and, in a sense, a part of the HIV scientific community.

Historically, medical information was solely the domain of physicians, healthcare professionals, and scientists. The doctor was in charge, and the patient submitted to the physician's recommendations and orders. Take, for instance, the term compliance. Fifteen years ago, doctors would prescribe a therapy and then monitor how *compliant* the patient was with respect to that therapy. By definition, to comply means to conform to someone's wishes. Simply put, the patient was expected to conform to the doctor's decision, regardless of his or her own wishes.

Times have changed, and today medicine is no longer just for the physician. People living with HIV are at the grassroots of a movement that has taken the hierarchy out of the doctor-patient relationship. Patients and doctors now work together as equals in developing care plans, assessing needs, and creating treatment regimes that meet the common goals of patient and medical professional. Take our example from the previous paragraph. Today, patients no longer comply with their doctors' wishes; they *adhere* to a given therapy. Webster's Online Dictionary defines the word adhere as the action of joining or uniting. Today doctors and patients unite or work together to develop care plans and medication therapies for the person living with HIV. This partnership is possible because of the determination and desire of patients to learn about their HIV. People living with HIV and AIDS are dedicated to the process of self-education.

1

But all that being said, does education improve prognosis and quality of life? The answer is a resounding *yes!* In fact, scientific studies have proven time and time again that educated and knowledgeable patients fare much better than those who aren't. In one study, researchers at RAND, a research institute in Santa Monica, California, found that the educated patient is much better able to adhere to treatment regimens than the patient with less education. Experts attribute this improved prognosis to the fact that greater understanding of a disease process contributes to an increased desire to take an active role in one's own healthcare. In stark contrast to twenty years ago, patients no longer submit to their doctors' wishes. Instead, they take an active role in their own care.

HIV is very complex. How is a lay person supposed to learn about and understand such a complicated condition? And what is the most effective way for a person to learn about their disease process? The effectiveness of any patient education tool depends on many factors, ranging from the educator's own experiences and qualifications to patients' preconceived ideas about their illness and their own health. But most important, the success of health education depends on the patient's willingness and ability to learn. Ideally, people living with HIV could sit down with a medical practitioner, nurse or other educator and learn about their disease process. Unfortunately, staffing shortages, financial factors, and time constraints put much of the education burden on the person living with the disease; in other words, it's all about self-education. So in order to self-educate properly, people need the right tools with which to learn. People need resources that are current, accurate and in a form that is conducive to learning. *Living with HIV: A Patient's Guide* is the tool people have been looking for.

Your desire and willingness to learn about your disease is evident by the fact you're reading this text. And you won't be disappointed. The following chapters will take you through the entire HIV lifespan—from prevention to diagnosis and beyond. HIV affects the entire person, both the physical and the emotional. This book provides you with the information you need to address both. Choosing a doctor can be confusing and frightening. This book will walk you through the process of finding a doctor that is right for you. Medications loom in the distance for some, and for others they're already part of the daily routine. This text will prepare you for medications, help you work through the side effects, improve your medication adherence, and help you assist your doctor in choosing the regimen that's right for you. And when the time comes for you to address the inevitability of any chronic illness, this book will walk you through end-of-life issues such as advanced directives, living wills, and hospice.

For those of you newly diagnosed, you're frightened of what the future holds. For those of you who have been living with HIV for years or decades, you need to take the next step in understanding your illness. And for those of you caring for a loved one, you want to be there for support when he or she needs you most. This book will help all of you achieve the educational goals you have set for yourself. You have in your hand a resource that will help you take control of your life and your illness. Knowledge is power, and having opened this text, you have taken a very important first step in living your life with HIV.

Now let's get started.

1

The History
of HIV and AIDS

In July 1981 millions of people around the world watched the royal wedding of Prince Charles and Lady Diana Spencer. That same year martial law was declared in Poland, the first IBM personal computer was introduced, and NASA launched the first space shuttle. While Pope John Paul II struggled for his life after an unsuccessful assassination attempt, small groups of gay men in New York and California were losing their battle with a rare and fatal form of cancer called Kaposi's sarcoma. Still others were presenting to emergency departments in Los Angeles and New York City with a seldom seen pneumonia called *Pneumocystis (carinii) jiroveci*. As people watched the nationally televised attempt on President Ronald Reagan's life, the greatest public health threat of the twentieth century was emerging, to the notice of almost no one.

HIV Is Older Than You Think

Publicly, the HIV/AIDS epidemic began in 1981. However, scientists now agree that HIV actually appeared decades earlier. The first theories suggested HIV was present in the late 1930s, a consequence of poorly conducted polio vaccine trials. Some even suggested HIV was the result of secret germ warfare research. But the most reliable evidence dates the first HIV and AIDS related illnesses to somewhere around 1959.

The presumed first victim of AIDS is thought to be a man from the Belgian Congo. Initially he presented to a local clinic with symptoms that resembled sickle cell anemia. Sickle cell is a hereditary blood disorder characterized by oddly shaped blood cells, a condition commonly found in the Congo at that time. Because of that fact, nobody questioned the diagnosis.

In the mid–1990s, in an effort to date the emergence of HIV and AIDS, leading HIV researcher David Ho and his colleagues at the Aaron Diamond Research Center examined blood samples taken from the man decades earlier.

The researchers found evidence of HIV, but what intrigued Ho was that the HIV found appeared to be an ancestor of the HIV infecting people in the 1990s. To Ho, this provided strong evidence that HIV entered the human species just prior to 1959, refuting earlier theories suggesting its emergence closer to 1935.

While we're fairly certain when HIV first infected man, no one knows for sure how. While scientists are certain HIV is a descendant of a Simian Immunodeficiency Virus (SIV), a virus found in monkeys, it's not entirely clear how the virus jumped from monkeys to humans. In 1995, scientists studied blood from a woman who died of AIDS and found her HIV to be a unique variant possessing characteristics of both HIV and SIV, suggesting that SIV somehow changes over time and becomes HIV. In African tribes, monkey meat is a large part of the diet. Experts theorize that eating the meat or brains of SIV infected monkeys introduced the virus into the human species, where it changed over time to become HIV, the virus that now runs rampant around the world.

AIDS Makes Its Worldwide Debut

Despite evidence that HIV was around in the late 1950s, the AIDS epidemic really didn't officially burst onto the scene until 1981. In June of that year a report from the Centers for Disease Control discussed an emerging epidemic among gay men, characterized by shortness of breath, chest pain, fevers and a productive cough requiring hospitalization. Bronchial biopsy of five patients confirmed the diagnosis: *pneumocystis (carinii) jiroveci pneumonia*, a rare but potentially fatal lung infection. What concerned experts was the fact that pneumocystis pneumonia occurred almost exclusively in people with severely weakened immune systems. The group of gay men presenting with pneumocystis had no previous history of illnesses that would weaken their immune systems. Experts also found that all the patients had CMV infections and thrush, both infections that mainly occur in people with very weak immune systems.

Another source of concern was the fact that all the patients involved were gay men, suggesting the cause of the weakened immune systems and the pneumocystis was related to sexual lifestyle or was sexually transmitted. This fact alone was especially concerning because the CDC realized that any disease transmitted sexually could potentially become a public health nightmare.

When news of the pneumocystis outbreak hit the *New York Times*, the public immediately made it an issue of morality because of its connection to the gay community. At that time, homosexuality already was a source of social stigma and prejudice. In the court of public opinion, the fact that a fatal, contagious, sexually transmitted disease had been linked to the gay population justified prejudice. People infected with the mysterious disease were immediately labeled as a risk to public safety and were deemed as sexual deviants, perverted, and immoral. Unlike other terminal illnesses that garner public support and empathy, HIV became the "gay plague," much like leprosy a century before. A combination of fear and ignorance gave birth to AIDS prejudice and discrimination.

The "Gay Cancer"

While the CDC struggled to find a cause for the sudden increase in pneumocystis among gay men, another concern arose among the same population. Kaposi's sarcoma (KS), a cancer normally seen in about 2 of every 3 million people, was appearing in young, gay men in alarming numbers. In a five week period in 1981, 41 cases of Kaposi's sarcoma were diagnosed, all of them in gay men. Most of the 41 would be dead within 24 months. Doctors investigating the outbreak found that all of the victims of KS had severely weakened immune systems, had reported having other infections (such as herpes and CMV), were recreational drug users, and admitted to having multiple sex partners. Again, the public made KS a morality issue and labeled it the "gay cancer," stereotyping gay men as promiscuous drug addicts and thereby furthering the discrimination against those living with AIDS.

The one saving grace for a gay man was that his lifestyle was private. Hiding one's sexuality, commonly referred to as "being in the closet," served as protection from the stereotypes and prejudices that faced gay men. That all changed with the emergence of KS. Characterized by dark lesions on the skin, men were identified as gay simply by the presence of KS lesions. The movie *Philadelphia* was based on such a premise. In the film, an attorney was fired, and his illness and sexuality were called into question, when his boss noticed the attorney's KS lesions. The movie's premise reflected real life. When the media made public the connection between KS and AIDS, men could no longer hide their sexual lifestyle or their illness. The dark lesions of KS became the face of AIDS.

The Term AIDS Is Born

Over the course of the next year, deaths related to pneumocystis and KS began to climb. And while an exact cause was still a mystery, the CDC determined that the mysterious illness was blood borne. It was in 1982 that the CDC renamed the disease Acquired Immune Deficiency Syndrome, or AIDS for short. While the media ran with AIDS-related stories almost every night, then–President Ronald Reagan had not yet commented on the emerging public health crisis. In fact, President Reagan's press secretary, Larry Speakes, made light of the illness at a press conference in 1982:

Q: Larry, does the President have any reaction to the announcement the Centers for Disease Control in Atlanta that AIDS is now an epidemic and has over 600 cases?

MR. SPEAKES: What's AIDS?

Q: Over a third of them have died. It's known as "gay plague." [Laughter] No, it is. I mean it's a pretty serious thing that one in every three people that get this has died. And I wondered if the President is aware of it?

MR. SPEAKES: I don't have it. Do you? [Laughter]

Q: No, I don't.

MR. SPEAKES: You didn't answer my question.

Q: Well, I just wondered, does the President...

MR. SPEAKES: How do you know? [Laughter]

Q: In other words, the White House looks on this as a great joke?

MR. SPEAKES: No, I don't know anything about it, Lester.

Q: Does the President, does anyone in the White House know about this epidemic, Larry?

MR. SPEAKES: I don't think so. I don't think there's been any...

Q: Nobody knows?

MR. SPEAKES: There has been no personal experience here, Lester.

Q: No, I mean, I thought you were keeping...

MR. SPEAKES: I checked thoroughly with Dr. Ruge this morning and he's had no [laughter] no patients suffering from AIDS or whatever it is.

Q: The President doesn't have gay plague, is that what you're saying or what?

MR. SPEAKES: No, I didn't say that.

Q: Didn't say that?

MR. SPEAKES: I thought I heard you on the State Department over there. Why didn't you stay there? [Laughter]

Q: Because I love you Larry, that's why. [Laughter]

MR. SPEAKES: Oh I see. Just don't put it in those terms, Lester. [Laughter]

Q: Oh, I retract that.

MR. SPEAKES: I hope so.

Q: It's too late.

While the government ignored the problem, a grassroots effort began, working to find research funding and to protect the rights of those with the new disease. One such group was the Gay Men's Health Crisis (GMHC). The group began with 80 men meeting at the home of author Larry Kramer to discuss the gay community's health crisis. Staffed entirely by volunteers, GMHC set up an AIDS hotline in the basement of its future director, Rodger McFarlane. In the first night of operation, the hotline received over 100 calls. It was obvious that that AIDS had reached epidemic proportions. The CDC agreed. By the end of 1982 they officially declared AIDS to be an epidemic.

A Cause Is Found ... but by Whom?

Over the next two years, work continued in an effort to find the cause of AIDS. Public concern rose when the CDC announced that, given the blood borne nature of AIDS, the donated blood supply may be unsafe. If true, AIDS would no longer be considered a disease limited to the gay community. This fact was reinforced with the announcement of a major outbreak of AIDS in Africa. But unlike the outbreak in the U.S., the African outbreak was found to be spread primarily by way of heterosexual contact. This marked the beginning of the AIDS crisis in Africa, as well as the safer sex movement in the western world.

A major breakthrough occurred in 1983 when Dr. Luc Montagnier of the Institut Pasteur in France announced that he and his colleagues found what they believed to be the virus responsible for AIDS. Human Immunodeficiency Virus or HIV, as it would be called, was a virus that damaged the immune system, weakening the body's defenses and making the body susceptible to infection. Experts were hopeful that the discovery of a cause would pave the way to a treatment and possibly a cure. But the discovery did create some controversy. A year after Institut Pasteur announced its discovery, Dr. Robert Gallo of the United States announced he too had discovered the virus responsible for AIDS. Gallo's research techniques came into question when accusations suggested that Gallo improperly used samples of HIV produced by Institut Pasteur en route to the discovery. Today, consensus among scientists is that Montagnier first discovered HIV, and it was Gallo who provided further evidence that the virus did indeed cause AIDS. The two groups continued to dispute each other's claim until 1985 when they agreed to share credit for the discovery.

Soon after the discovery of HIV, the Food and Drug Administration (FDA) approved a test that detected antibodies to the virus, indicating infection. This provided a method that allowed doctors to identify patients infected with HIV prior to them exhibiting any signs of illness or infection. The new test was an important step in fighting the spread of AIDS. Blood banks could test their supplies to assure they were HIV free, and people infected could be diagnosed earlier, allowing for treatment that improved quality of life.

A cause had been determined, and a test to detect that cause had been developed. All that was needed was an effective treatment. While the world awaited such a breakthrough, people continued to die in alarming numbers. AIDS became a household word in 1985 with the diagnosis of actor Rock Hudson. His announcement that he had AIDS and was going to France to seek experimental treatment put a familiar face on the epidemic. His death later that year made the list of the *Wall Street Journal*'s most significant stories in its 100 year history.

Finally ... a Treatment

Despite $1.3 billion being invested annually in HIV research, a cure was still nowhere to be found. The development of an HIV vaccine was as remote as a cure, so in an effort to improve prognosis and to lengthen lives, treatment for the disease became an urgent priority. By an Executive order, the United States closed its borders to HIV infected immigrants and travelers by 1985. While President Reagan finally discussed the AIDS crisis, negative public opinion regarding the Administration's handling of the AIDS epidemic continued to mount. The vice president at the time, George Bush, suggested the U.S. should institute mandatory HIV testing of its citizens in hopes of putting a halt to the illness's rapid spread. Prejudice, ignorance and fear had reached unprecedented levels with the burning of a Florida home in an attempt to drive the family and their two HIV-infected sons from the neighborhood. Both sons contracted HIV from tainted blood products received as part of their treatment for hemophilia. To their neighbors, why they were HIV infected was not important. The fact they were infected with HIV made them a threat to those who weren't — an all too common and very dangerous way of thinking in the United States in the post–AIDS era.

The first glimmer of hope arrived in 1987 when drug manufacturer Glaxo-SmithKline (Glaxo-Wellcome at the time) gained FDA approval for the world's first drug to treat HIV. Zidovudine, or AZT, as it became known, was to be given as a 400mg dose taken every four hours around the clock. Twenty years earlier, AZT was studied as an anti-cancer drug, but studies were halted because the drug showed little promise due to its high rate of toxicity and side effects. Yet, short term studies in HIV patients showed dramatic results. While side effects such as low blood count (anemia) were common, patient prognosis did improve. So, despite side effects and issues of toxicity, Glaxo stopped trials early and sought approval from the FDA.

While the development of an HIV medication was a wonderful step forward, the approval of AZT was not without difficulty. First, GlaxoWellcome was publicly blasted for what the HIV community called "price gouging," with its $7000-per-year AZT price tag. It took two years and intense pressure by HIV activist groups for Glaxo to reduce the price of AZT by 20 percent in 1989. The second controversy questioned the effectiveness and safety of AZT therapy. Some groups theorized that it was AZT itself that caused AIDS, not HIV. Stories of toxic side effects and birth defects were common, adding fuel to the AZT controversy. Even today, certain groups continue to insist AZT is the killer, not HIV or AIDS. But despite the controversy, AZT was widely prescribed and did show promising results, at least in the short term.

Given the positive results among those taking AZT, a new emphasis on HIV drug development was born. The FDA process for approving new drugs normally took years, but in the case of people infected with HIV, most didn't have years to wait. Pressured by AIDS activist groups like Act Up, the FDA announced a rapid drug approval system for HIV meds, shaving at least two years off the approval process.

Does Anyone Notice?

As the epidemic raged on, those in the HIV community struggled to get the world to notice what was happening. The AIDS Memorial Quilt was started as a tribute to those who lost their struggle against HIV/AIDS. Authors and playwrights tried to explain HIV and AIDS through such works as *And the Band Played On* and *The Normal Heart.* Those dying from HIV were no longer faceless strangers. Pianist and song writer Liberace, actress Amanda Blake, and Michael Bennett, director of the Broadway play *Chorus Line*, all fell victim to AIDS.

Politicians of the time, while slow to react to the epidemic, did realize what dangerous prejudice and discrimination was occurring against those living with HIV. A 1988 law made it illegal to discriminate against anyone infected with HIV. It was a small step in the right direction, but, unfortunately, discrimination and prejudice continued.

In 1988, C. Everett Koop, surgeon general of the United States, released a report emphasizing the need for sex education in order to slow the spread of HIV. To that end, the U.S. Department of Health and Human Services mailed out 107 million copies of its booklet *Understanding AIDS* in hopes that a better understanding of HIV and AIDS would slow the spread of the disease through safer sex, and at the same time would quell the prejudice, discrimination and fear directed at those living with HIV. But, unfortunately, like attempts before this one, it had little effect on the public's opinion of people living with HIV.

The Courage of Ryan White

The 1990s began with a public apology from Ronald Reagan for his neglect of HIV and AIDS during his presidency. In a public service announcement to benefit the Pediatric AIDS Foundation, Reagan called for compassion and understanding for those living with AIDS. One of those people Reagan referred to was Ryan White. A teenage boy who contracted HIV/AIDS through blood products he received to treat his hemophilia, Ryan White experienced AIDS prejudice and hatred first hand. He and his family fought the Kokomo, Indiana, school board to allow Ryan to attend public school. Because of ignorance and fear, the people of Kokomo showed little support for Ryan's cause. Students vandalized his locker, townspeople vandalized the White's home, and local restaurants threw away the dishes from which he and his family ate. After a gunshot was fired into their living room, the Whites moved to Cicero, Indiana, where they were welcomed with open arms. Ryan attended public school, got his drivers permit, and became an example of hope and courage for the entire HIV community. Ryan White died in 1990, but his struggle was not forgotten. Later that year, the United States Congress passed the Ryan White Care Act, providing funds for HIV care and prevention. Today the act remains one of the most important sources of HIV care funding in the world.

A Change of Course

The year 1991 saw the re-emergence of an old public health nemesis. Tuberculosis, or TB, as it is called, resurfaced after years of being controlled through organized testing and the development of antibiotics such as streptomycin. At one time, hospitals had TB wards, isolating those infected. TB sanitariums were commonplace in large urban areas. In fact, TB was once the leading cause of death in the U.S. But with the development of antibiotics, the deaths decreased dramatically, and new infections were all but eliminated. But with the emergence of AIDS, people whose immune systems were weakened by HIV became a high risk for TB. New cases started to emerge, especially in urban centers, among the homeless and in the prison system. Today, yearly TB screenings are a standard of care for people living with HIV.

President George Bush continued the policies of his predecessor. Despite a recommendation to the contrary from his secretary of health, Louis Sullivan, Bush continued the ban on the immigration of HIV positive people. And while the Ryan White Care Act authorized $881 million of emergency relief for those cities hit hardest by HIV and AIDS, the administration eventually allocated only $350 million. But change was in the wind. Presidential candidate Bill Clinton promised full funding of the Ryan White Care Act, a lifting of the immigration ban, and the naming of an HIV "Czar" whose sole purpose was to address the problem of AIDS. Clinton's election in 1992 was seen by many as a positive step in the fight against HIV and AIDS.

On the treatment front, the choices of HIV medications were increasing. In a 24 month period between 1991 and 1994, the drugs Videx, Hivid, and Zerit were all approved by the FDA. Hivid was the first to be approved for use in combination with AZT. Study data made it clear that multiple drug therapy was superior to single drug therapy. By 1993, experts reported that patients were beginning to show resistance to the drug AZT, especially among those who used AZT alone. The consensus among HIV experts was that multiple drug therapy would be stronger and more effective, and would delay resistance to the medications. Their hypothesis was supported when, later that year, studies determined that AZT taken alone early in the course of infection did nothing to improve long-term prognosis or slow the progression to AIDS. In fact, that year's IX International Conference on AIDS made it clear that neither AZT nor any of the available antiretroviral drugs were useful for early treatment. The announcement couldn't come at a worse time. The statistics were quite sobering. By the end of 1993, almost 400,000 people had been infected since the epidemic began, and almost 200,000 of those had died.

AIDS was quickly garnering the attention of Hollywood. In response to the deaths of entertainers such as Rock Hudson, Amanda Blake, and Rudolph Nureyev, Hollywood producers, writers, and entertainers rallied to raise money and awareness. In September 1993, HBO premiered its film adaptation of the Randy Shilts novel *And the Band Played On*. In December, Tom Hanks starred in the movie *Philadelphia*, a story of an attorney fired by his firm because of HIV. Hanks won the Best Actor Oscar for his role as the attorney, yet some critics in the gay and HIV community claimed that his character fell short because the film lacked outward signs of affection normally found in gay relationships. Regardless, the Hollywood support was beginning to pay off in terms of money and awareness.

Bring Out the Big Guns — the Protease Inhibitor

An HIV drug is classed according to where in the HIV life cycle the medication has its intended effect. Prior to 1995, only one drug class was available, the nucleoside reverse transcriptase inhibitors (NRTI). That meant only one place in the life cycle could be attacked. Regimens consisting of two NRTIs were used occasionally, but most often treatment consisted of only one drug. Unfortunately, studies were beginning to reveal that one-drug treatment, or monotherapy, as it was called, was not strong enough to suppress HIV reproduction for very long. In addition, drug resistance developed quickly, eventually making the medications ineffective. And the most worrisome issue surrounding monotherapy was that resistance to one NRTI meant resistance to all drugs in that class. It was evident that patients would run out of drug choices very quickly. A new and stronger class of drug was needed badly. As the world waited for this new class, AIDS had become the leading cause of death in Americans 25 to 44 years of age.

The FDA recognized the urgent need for new treatments. In a record 97 days, the drug manufacturer Roche received FDA approval for a new class of HIV medication, the protease inhibitor (PI). The first in this class was the drug Saquinavir. It attacked HIV at an entirely different place in the life cycle than existing drugs available at the time. With the addition of PIs, HIV could be attacked on two fronts, which meant treatments were more effective and lasted longer. Protease inhibitors like Saquinavir made more powerful "drug cocktails" possible. The downside to PI-containing cocktails was that the regimens had large pill burdens and severe side effects. Still, the advent of the protease inhibitor prompted some media sources to report that the PI was the AIDS breakthrough that could spell the end of the epidemic.

More Meds, but Testing and Prevention Become Key

While preliminary results of combination therapy looked promising, experts agreed that the key to controlling the epidemic was testing and prevention. Prevention education, once generalized to target the public as a whole, was being retooled to address specific populations. Educators found that prevention messages were better received if they "spoke" to the intended population. For example, a prevention message targeted to gay white men may not be well received by bisexual black men unwilling to admit they had sex with other men. Many felt this small change was a very important step forward in HIV/AIDS education.

From the beginning of the epidemic, experts have realized the importance of early diagnosis through HIV testing. Unfortunately, because of the stigma and prejudices associated with AIDS, a large share of the population was reluctant to get tested. People feared that even being tested would bring on the same discrimination and prejudices faced by those people living with the infection. In response, HIV test manufacturers worked to develop a test that would alleviate some of those fears. In 1996 the FDA approved the first home test kit for HIV. Experts hoped that the anonymity of home testing would encourage people to get tested and learn their status. Unfortunately, it was discovered many years later that not all home test kits were created equal. Doubts about accuracy and reliability surfaced, and the home test kit idea suffered. While still available, home tests never became a primary mode of HIV testing.

Advances in HIV science continued in 1996. A third class of HIV medication, the non-nucleoside reverse transcriptase inhibitors (NNRTI), gained FDA approval, providing one more weapon against HIV. A third angle of attack meant regimens were more powerful and lasted longer. The timing was perfect. Studies showed that more than 14 percent of all people taking existing HIV medications were exhibiting signs of HIV resistance. Experts began to worry that if the trend continued there would eventually be no means to treat HIV. Fear of an epidemic similar to what was happening in Africa at the time sent chills through the HIV scientific community. The addition of Roxanne Laboratories' new NNRTI, Nevirapine, was reason for hope. The drug added a new layer to HIV treatment, again making regimens more powerful and more effective. At about the same time, a new technology made it possible for doctors to monitor the fight against the virus. By the end of 1996, the FDA had approved for use the world's first HIV viral load, allowing doctors to quantify how well new drug combinations were suppressing HIV.

Since the epidemic began, what most people, scientific and general public alike, considered the Holy Grail of HIV research was the HIV vaccine. Like the polio vaccine decades before, people envisioned an HIV vaccine that would offer permanent protection against AIDS. What many felt could be the realization of that dream was the announcement of the first human tests of an HIV

vaccine in 1996. Over 5000 people from across the U.S. took that first coura-
geous step by volunteering to receive the new vaccine. While hopes were high,
researchers cautioned that a usable, effective HIV vaccine could still be decades
away.

More Sobering Statistics

As the end of the twentieth century neared, HIV/AIDS statistics from
around the world did little to instill hope in those fighting the disease. By the
year 2000, women and minorities were bearing the brunt of the HIV epidemic.
AIDS had become the leading cause of death in women 25 to 44 years old, and
African Americans accounted for 49 percent of AIDS deaths in the United
States. And even with the emphasis on testing, New York City officials estimated
that nearly 70,000 people were unaware they were HIV infected, a large percentage of those minorities. Public health experts feared that this fact would
eventually translate into a geometric increase in new HIV infection numbers
among minorities, a potential disaster that would eventually repeat itself in
every large urban area in the United States.

While not all the news was bad, even the good news was problematic in
some respects. From 1998 through 2001, deaths related to AIDS steadily declined
from a peak of almost 18,000 to a low of just under 9000. The consensus was
that the declining death rate was the result of more powerful and effective HIV
medications. On the surface, this would appear to be very good news. Yet new
HIV infections were on the rise, and there was a theory why. The success of
HIV medications was making HIV a long-term, manageable condition, as
opposed to the death sentence it once was. Experts feared the successes were
diminishing the public's appreciation of the seriousness of HIV, leading to an
increase in high risk behaviors such as unprotected sex. This, in turn, led to
the increase in new infections.

The New Century Arrives

As the new century arrived, scientists from around the world gathered in
Durban, South Africa, epicenter of the HIV epidemic, for the XIII International AIDS Conference. Over 12,000 participants witnessed the devastation of
AIDS first hand, prompting 5000 doctors to sign the Durban Declaration, a document of overwhelming affirmation that HIV causes AIDS.

On the medication front, the age-old problem of medication adherence
was being addressed with the development of many once-a-day therapies with
diminishing pill burden. Experts had found that HIV drugs, while very effec-

tive, were prone to resistance. A major cause of drugs becoming ineffective was poor regimen adherence. Medications not taken consistently, and doses missed or portions of multiple drug regimens omitted due to side effects, caused HIV to adapt and mutate, eventually making the drug regimen ineffective. In an effort to improve adherence and thereby reduce the incidence of mutation and resistance, drug manufacturers began combining existing medications into new combination drugs. For instance, Combivir, the combination of AZT and Epivir, reduced a two-drug therapy from four pills each day to two. Trizivir, the combination of AZT, Epivir, and Ziagen, reduced a three-drug regimen from six pills each day to two. By decreasing the number of pills required each day, adherence would improve, the incidence of mutation and resistance would decrease, and therapies would be more effective for longer periods of time.

Medication improvements were not limited to NRTIs and NNRTIs. Protease inhibitors, notorious for very large pill burdens taken several times each day, were being improved as well. For instance, the drugs Norvir and Lopinavir were combined into the drug Kaletra, allowing the drug to be taken twice each day and diminishing the Norvir side effects that negatively impacted medication adherence in the past. The 2003 FDA approval of the PI Reyataz made it possible for doctors to prescribe the most powerful class of HIV drug as two capsules once each day. An excellent example of PI improvement came in 2003 with the release of Lexiva. By changing the formulation of the existing drug Amprenavir to create Lexiva, pill burden was decreased from sixteen pills each day to four.

Drug manufacturers realized that decreasing the number of pills alone was not enough to significantly improve adherence. Some drugs, while very effective, were difficult to take because of side effects. Something had to be done to make drugs more palatable. A perfect example of advances made in drug formulation was the medication Videx EC. The drug Videx had been part of drug regimens for several years. Consisting of four wafers that had to be chewed or dissolved in liquid, Videx was almost impossible to take consistently due to the poor taste and the vomiting it frequently caused. To address the problem, the manufacturer reformulated the drug into Videx EC, a capsule that could be taken once daily. This change in formulation decreased the side effects, and made the drug much easier to take — swallowing one capsule, as opposed to chewing or dissolving four wafers. This greatly improved adherence to the drug, making it one of the key medications used to treat HIV in 2004.

Another drug known for its severe side effects was Norvir. Taken as six capsules twice each day, Norvir caused severe gastrointestinal side effects, making adherence very difficult. However, researchers found that in small doses, Norvir improved the effect of other medications and was much more tolerable. In response to this finding, doctors began to prescribe Norvir as a *boosting* agent for other PIs, most often in doses as small as one capsule per day. This improved adherence and at the same time strengthened regimens.

Where Are We Now?

After twenty plus years, and despite advances in treatment access, medication development, adherence tools, and education and prevention, the HIV epidemic continues. The number of new infections in the United States remains at about 56,000 each year, while in other parts of the world, such as Asia, India, and Russia, the rates of new infection is much higher. In Africa, the HIV epidemic has caused financial hardship, has orphaned millions of children, and has brought about negative population growth in many areas.

The key to slowing the spread of HIV is easy access to health care and medications. Unfortunately, many countries lack the resources to treat their population. The United States has pledged $50 billion globally for treatment, education, and prevention, but many feel this is not nearly enough. At the same time, drug manufacturers are beginning to ease their strict policies regarding generic formulations of HIV medications in an attempt to improve medication access. For instance, drug manufacturer Boehringer Ingelheim has taken a first step, allowing a South African drug company to make a generic version of the drug Viramune, while Barr Laboratories has gained FDA approval for its generic form of Videx EC.

A constant concern within the HIV community and for HIV caregivers is funding. The Ryan White CARE Act was reauthorized in 2000 and again in 2006, but since that time seven of the nine U.S. cities receiving Title I funding under the CARE Act have experienced significant funding cuts. In addition, those programs not experiencing funding cuts have been *flat funded*. Simply put, each program receives a predetermined amount of money to run their program. While the costs of running their program increase, the amount of funding stays the same. Eventually, to maintain their program, budget cuts are necessary.

Debate continues on how best to fight the spread of HIV. While federal funding has been slowly shifted from prevention programs to treatment programs, prevention education has taken on political tones. Some lawmakers have made HIV education a morality issue. The Bush Administration has made it clear that prevention should be abstinence-based, allocating almost one third of its prevention budget to abstinence training. Despite studies confirming abstinence education is not the most effective way to slow the spread of HIV, the CDC was ordered to remove condom educational materials from its website, and to replace it with abstinence educational material. After public and scientific outcry, the CDC returned the condom information in a watered down format, deemphasizing the effectiveness of condom use in preventing pregnancy and sexually transmitted diseases.

The benefit and morality of condoms was not the only source of controversy. Sharing needles and syringes among injection drug users is a major source of HIV transmission. Studies have shown that providing clean needles and syringes through needle exchange programs has decreased transmission significantly. Yet, debate continues surrounding who should fund such programs. Current laws prohibit federal funding of such programs, so agencies are left to find private funding, a task made much more difficult in times of economic troubles.

Since the year 2000, three new drug classes have been added: nucleotide reverse transcriptase inhibitors, the first of which is the oral drug Viread (tenofovir); integrase inhibitors, with the first drug in the class being Isentress (raltegravir); and entry inhibitors, represented by the two drugs Selzentry (maraviroc) and the injectable medication Fuzeon (enfuvirtide). These drugs have added to the arsenal of weapons available to practitioners. The emphasis on adherence and drug improvement continues with the FDA's announcement that combination drugs, such as the new combinations Truvada (tenofovir + emtricitabine), Atripla (efavirenz+tenofovir+emtricitabine) and Epzicom (lamivudine+abacavir), can move through the drug approval process much quicker. The *accelerated track system* was created by the FDA in an effort to get new, improved HIV meds to the public in much less time. Meanwhile, vaccine research continues, but significant progress is still nowhere in sight. In fact, HIV vaccine researcher VaxGen announced in 2004 that its trial vaccine, AIDSVax, proved ineffective in its initial testing of 5400 participants.

What Does the Future Hold?

Each year that passes brings new advances in the treatment of HIV and AIDS. Treatment guidelines, reviewed annually, now recommend that medications should be started sooner rather than later, but not quite as early as the "hit 'em early and hit 'em hard" mentality of several years ago. Work continues on an HIV vaccine, improving adherence by simplifying medication regimens, and understanding the long term effects of HIV medications. Trials are moving forward on a new class of HIV medication, one that attacks HIV during its maturation process. When perfected, this class would interfere with the virus's ability to mature and reproduce. Finally, work continues in hopes of gaining a better understanding of HIV's long-term effects.

So the learning process continues for those treating the disease, as well as for those living with HIV and AIDS. Now you know the history of the disease you're fighting. You know where we've been, and you've had a glimpse of where we're going. But that's just the beginning.

2

HIV Prevention and Testing

The first step in slowing the HIV epidemic is prevention. In fact, HIV is a preventable disease — if the proper precautions are taken. Since the onset of the epidemic, prevention efforts have significantly affected the spread of HIV. We need only to look at Africa to see what would be if not for prevention education. In 2002, David Holtgrave, a health policy educator at Emory University, published a report that discussed the impact prevention has had on the epidemic in the United States. By looking at infection rates in Africa, Holtgrave was able to calculate how the HIV picture would look today in the U.S. if not for the prevention efforts that have been in place for the last two decades. The numbers are frightening. Holtgrave has estimated that as many as 1.5 million more people in the United States would be infected today if not for HIV prevention.

Effective prevention starts with education. The public needs to know how HIV is transmitted, what behaviors increase the risk of transmission, and what steps can be taken to reduce the risk of acquiring HIV infection. Let's start by reviewing how HIV is spread from person to person.

Conditions Needed for HIV Transmission

Three conditions must be met for HIV transmission to occur. First, HIV must be present in the blood or bodily fluids involved in the exposure. Second, HIV must be in sufficient quantities to cause infection. In blood, HIV is very concentrated, so a very small amount of blood can infect. In other bodily fluids, such has semen, HIV is less concentrated, so the amount needed for transmission is greater. Finally, HIV must make its way into the bloodstream. HIV on the surface of unbroken skin is not going to infect because the virus can't make it to the blood stream. On the other hand, mucous membranes or open wounds give HIV access to the bloodstream, making transmission more likely.

Where in the Body Is HIV Located?

All bodily fluids contain HIV, but only some in concentrations great enough to cause HIV transmission. Table 1 illustrates which fluids do and do not transmit HIV.

TABLE 1	
Fluids That Transmit HIV	*Fluids That Don't Transmit HIV*
Blood (Including Menstrual Blood)	Saliva
Semen	Tears
Vaginal and Rectal Secretions	Sweat
Breast Milk	Urine
Pre-cum	Feces

Keep in mind that while these fluids do not cause HIV infection, they can transmit other diseases, such as Hepatitis B and Hepatitis C.

Transmission Routes

SEXUAL TRANSMISSION

The most common means of transmitting HIV is through sexual contact between two men, two women, or a man and a woman. Studies confirm that the transmission of HIV between men who have sex with other men is most frequently due to unprotected anal intercourse. The receptive partner ("the bottom") is at higher risk than the inserting partner ("the top"). The mucous membranes that make up the lining of the rectum provide a large surface for exposure to infected bodily fluids, such as semen. Rectal trauma from anal intercourse results in tears and tissue damage that make it easier for HIV to enter the blood stream. The inserting partner can also be infected by exposure to rectal secretions and blood from rectal trauma.

The same mechanisms of infection hold true for vaginal intercourse. The mucous membranes of the vagina and cervix provide a large area where transmission can occur. Trauma to vaginal tissue increases the risk of transmission. At one time, it was hypothesized that HIV was more easily transmitted from male to female than from female to male. However, recent studies indicate that in the absence of special circumstances, such as IV drug use, the transmission risk from male to female is about the same as from female to male. There is also evidence that transmission from female to female can occur, but at a very low incidence. The most common means of transmission in this scenario is through the sharing of sex toys or through oral contact with infected bodily fluids. Transmission during oral sexual contact is much less common but can occur. Oral exposure to infected semen, vaginal secretions or rectal secretions has been known to transmit HIV; however, the risk is much lower than with vaginal or anal intercourse.

NEEDLES

The accidental injection of infected blood is a more effective means of HIV transmission than even sexual intercourse. In such places as Africa, sex between a man and woman is the most common means of HIV transmission. But outside of Africa, sharing needles among injection drug users plays a major role in the spread of HIV. As part of the process of injecting drugs, users pull infected blood into their needle and syringe. That needle and syringe is then used by another person, who injects the infected blood, along with the drug, into his or her blood stream. This process repeats itself over and over, leaving new HIV infections in its wake.

Another source of HIV transmission seen primarily in the healthcare industry is accidental needle sticks. Some sources estimate that more than 600,000 accidental needle sticks occur each year. While the Centers for Disease Control (CDC) reports less than 100 known cases of HIV transmission by accidental needle stick, the numbers for other blood borne diseases, such as Hepatitis C, are far greater. Hollow-bore needles used to draw blood or give injections carry the highest degree of risk. In an attempt to decrease the number of accidental needle sticks, there are efforts at the federal as well as state levels to mandate hospitals and medical practices to use safety needles to protect their workers.

FROM MOTHER TO BABY

HIV is spread from a woman to her baby in two ways. *Vertical transmission,* or transmission from an infected pregnant woman to her unborn child, can occur during pregnancy or during delivery. Exposure to infected blood or amniotic fluids while in the uterus or during a vaginal delivery provides the route by which HIV enters the baby's bloodstream. HIV transmission in this manner is very efficient, affecting about one in four births without proper treatment before, during and after delivery. To further reduce the risk of transmission, surgical delivery of the baby is far more common than vaginal delivery, thereby reducing the baby's exposure to the HIV-infected fluids of childbirth. Unfortunately, the methods used to achieve this low rate of infection are not readily available to women and babies in such places as Sub-Saharan Africa, fueling the raging epidemic in the Third World.

Another way in which newborns are exposed to HIV is from breast milk during breast feeding. In fact, breast feeding carries an extremely high risk of transmission — somewhere between 25 and 30 percent. Because of the high risk, HIV positive mothers are cautioned not to breast feed or manually express breast milk to feed their baby. The African epidemic continues in part because breast milk is the primary source of nourishment for newborn children in that country.

HIV-INFECTED BLOOD PRODUCTS

Since 1985, blood products have been thoroughly screened for HIV, virtually eliminating transmission of HIV through infected blood products. While the chance of infection from blood products is remote, the risk still exists. For instance, a person infected with HIV immediately prior to donating blood could donate blood that tests HIV-antibody negative but still carries the virus. During the "window" between HIV infection and HIV antibody production by the immune system, blood would test negative but would still be infectious. Keep in mind that this scenario is extremely rare, and infection in this manner virtually never happens.

There is, however, a large segment of the HIV population that acquired the disease through infected blood products. Hemophilia is a genetic disorder characterized by the absence of blood clotting factors. Daily infusion of donated clotting factor is the treatment for the disease. Prior to testing of donated blood, thousands of people with hemophilia were infected with HIV by the very blood products they infused to save their lives. Today, however, the transmission of HIV infection through infused blood products has been all but eliminated. Table 2 summarizes the HIV transmission routes.

TABLE 2

Sexual Transmission	Needles / Needle Sticks	Mother to Baby	Blood Products
Anal (Male-Male & Male-Female)	Sharing Needles While Injecting Drugs	During Pregnancy	Virtually Eliminated (Since Testing Started in 1985)
Vaginal	Accidental Needle Stick (Typically on the Job)	During Delivery	6,000–10,000 Hemophiliacs Infected (Due to Contaminated Blood Scandal)
Oral (Male-Male; Male-Female; Female-Male)		During Breastfeeding	

Now we know how HIV spreads from person to person. Let's take a look at how the spread of HIV can be prevented.

HIV Prevention Basics

HIV prevention addresses all three primary modes of transmission: sexual, needle sharing, and vertical transmission. Before discussing specific prevention techniques, let's take a look at a major theory in prevention education — the theory of *risk and harm rezduction*.

RISK REDUCTION

Early in the epidemic, prevention messages concentrated on teaching individuals how to avoid behaviors that lead to negative consequences. For instance, counselors instructed their clients to stop having sex with prostitutes in order to eliminate the risk of acquiring HIV. This prevention message ignores the effect certain personality traits have on a person's ability to do what's in their own best interest. Such educational approaches have proved ineffective for people fighting drug and alcohol addiction, as well as for those engaging in risky sexual behavior. Despite the risks, these people knowingly continue to engage in high-risk behavior. In order for prevention efforts to be effective, prevention specialists must consider these personality traits when developing their prevention tools and plans.

Risk reduction is a concept that considers personality traits when developing a holistic approach to HIV prevention. It takes into consideration the reality of human behavior. For example, teaching sexual abstinence as the only HIV prevention technique ignores the reality that a high percentage of teens will have sex despite the risks. Using risk reduction, teens are taught about abstinence as well as the proper way to use condoms in the event they do decide to have sex.

Risk reduction requires education, self assessment and behavior modification. The risk reduction model consists of four stages:

- **Labeling**—an individual must be able to assess and recognize his or her at-risk behavior. For instance, a person at this stage would say, "I know unprotected sex is unsafe."
- **Commitment**—an individual makes a commitment to certain goals that will diminish his or her risk of HIV. For instance, a person at this stage would say, "I will use a condom each time I have sex."
- **Enactment**—an individual has achieved behavioral change by removing barriers. A person at this stage would say, "I have discussed with my partner the importance of condoms, and we agree that we will use them each time we have sex."
- **Maintenance**—an individual sustains risk-reducing behavior. An individual at this stage would say, "Condoms are second nature to me now."

The term *safer sex* is a product of the risk reduction concept. Any sexual behavior can be unsafe. Safer sex refers to adjusting sexual behaviors in order to reduce risks associated with sexual activity. There are no 100 percent safe sex techniques, therefore the outdated term safe sex may be misleading to some and, in fact, may lead to high-risk behaviors. For instance, at one time oral sex was thought to be "safe." Many engaged in high-risk oral sex, unaware that it, too, carried some degree of risk. On the other hand, safer sex education assumes oral sex can be unsafe and teaches techniques to minimize the risk — thus, "safer sex."

SAFER SEX METHODS

There are several methods couples can employ to decrease the risk of HIV transmission. The most important thing is for couples to discuss safer sex prior to sexual activity. Trying to discuss safer sex in the "heat of the moment" is very difficult and most often not very effective. Discussions should be honest and frank. Being sexually intimate with a partner for the first time can be scary. Discussing the emotional and physical risks of sex and how to prevent those risks can be empowering and actually makes sex a more intense, enjoyable experience by creating an emotional understanding between the two partners. Remember, practicing safer sex does not mean eliminating sex from your life. It means being smart, minimizing risk, and staying healthy.

Abstinence

Abstinence is the voluntary choice to refrain from sexual activity and is the only safer sex method that is 100 percent effective in preventing HIV. Abstinence does not mean the absence of sexual intimacy, however. Non-coital forms of sexual intimacy include holding hands, hugging, and kissing, as well as petting, mutual masturbation, and the use of stimulating devices such as vibrators, which can be enjoyable alternatives to intercourse. Keep in mind that while abstinence is an effective means of safer sex, if may be impractical for some and very difficult to maintain over the course of an intimate relationship.

Condoms

Condoms are sheaths of thin latex or plastic that are placed on an erect penis prior to sexual intercourse. To be effective, condoms must be worn during sex and removed immediately after ejaculation. Condoms must be used during any oral, vaginal, or anal sexual contact. While using condoms, some very important points must be kept in mind.

- Condoms can break due to friction during sex, resulting in leakage of semen. To reduce the risk of this occurring, a generous amount of water soluble lubricant should be used. Oil-based lubricants such as petroleum jelly will weaken a condom and should never be used.
- Because it increases friction, two condoms should not be worn at the same time.
- An erect penis can leak pre-seminal fluid (precum) before ejaculation. This fluid can contain HIV. For this reason, condoms must be applied prior to any sexual contact.
- Condoms must be removed and discarded immediately after ejaculation. Never reuse a condom.

- For those people with latex allergies, non-latex, polyurethane condoms can be used. Keep in mind that sheepskin condoms have micro pores larger than HIV, allowing the virus to penetrate the condom. Consequently, they do not protect against HIV transmission and should never be used.
- Spermacides, such as nonoxynol-9, actually increases the risk of HIV transmission by irritating mucous membranes, allowing HIV to enter the bloodstream. For this reason spermacides should never be considered as protection against HIV.

The Female Condom

The *female condom* is a polyurethane pouch about seven inches in length worn by a woman during sex. It has a flexible ring on each end — one holds the condom against the cervix, and one holds the condom outside of the vagina. There is silicone lubricant on the inside of the condom to reduce friction, decreasing the risk of breakage during sex. The female condom is the only female-controlled device that offers protection against HIV. There are a few important points to keep in mind when using the female condom.

- Used correctly, the female condom is 79 percent to 95 percent effective in preventing HIV.
- The female condom can be put in place up to eight hours prior to sexual activity.
- Because friction can break condoms, a female condom and male condom should not be used at the same time.
- The female condom must be held in place during intercourse to prevent accidental displacement.
- After ejaculation, carefully remove the female condom and discard. Never reuse a female condom.

Dental Dams

Dental dams are rectangular squares of latex that are used during oral-vaginal and oral-anal sex. During sex, dams are stretched across the genitals to prevent bodily secretions from coming in contact with the mucous membranes of the mouth. While effective, dental dams can be a bit cumbersome and difficult to hold in place. A small amount of water soluble lubricant applied to the genital side of the dam can help keep them in place. After sex, they should be discarded and should never be reused.

PREVENTING PREGNANCY DOESN'T MEAN SAFER SEX

Regardless of their effectiveness in preventing pregnancy, there are several birth control methods that do nothing to protect the user from HIV. These tools should not be used to prevent HIV transmission.

- Diaphragms
- Intrauterine devices (IUDs)
- Birth control pills
- Hormonal implants and injections
- Spermacides
- Withdrawal
- Surgical sterilization of men or women

PREVENTING MOTHER TO BABY TRANSMISSION

Vertical Transmission

The HIV epidemic rages out of control in much of Africa in part due to the high incidence of infected pregnant women passing HIV to their unborn children. In the absence of medical care, this mode of transmission occurs in about one out of every four pregnancies. However, in the western world, advances in HIV treatment have nearly eliminated vertical transmission, decreasing the incidence to about 3 percent. The keys to this success include early diagnosis through aggressive screening programs, regular obstetrical care, and HIV treatment for the mother during pregnancy and delivery, and treatment for the newborn baby after delivery.

Breast Feeding

About 25 percent of all babies breast fed by an HIV infected woman will acquire the disease. In fact, the risk is even greater if mom is newly infected while she is breastfeeding. So in order to eliminate this transmission route, HIV infected women should never breast feed. In parts of the world where bottle feeding is available, this is a relatively simple solution. But in poorer regions such as Africa, the lack of financial resources, commercial formulas, and clean water makes bottle feeding impossible and HIV prevention very difficult, fueling an already out of control epidemic.

SHARING NEEDLES AND INJECTING DRUGS

Outside of sexual contact, needle sharing among injection drug users is the most common means of HIV transmission. Therefore, in order to significantly slow the spread of HIV, needle sharing must be eliminated, ideally by halting injection drug use. However, as our discussion of risk reduction revealed, human behavior and certain personality traits makes eliminating substance use impossible. A more realistic approach is to treat those who want treatment for their substance use and to reduce the risk for those who feel they need to continue injecting drugs.

Risk Reduction — Needle Exchange

Risk reduction takes a realistic approach to preventing the spread of HIV among drug users. One type of risk reduction is needle exchange. Community prevention agencies make sterile syringes and needles available in the community, exchanging them for used needles and syringes. Needle exchange is gaining popularity among prevention specialists as a proven method of HIV prevention. Unfortunately, needle exchange is a politically controversial subject. Opponents of needle exchange fear that making clean needles available to intravenous drug users facilitates further drug use. Political opponents have also made needle exchange a morality issue, refusing to fund a program that would supply the tools that support illegal drug habits.

Despite protests from opponents of needle exchange, it is a proven method of decreasing HIV infection among those who share needles. Exchanging used needles for clean ones eliminates the need to share needles, which in turn decreases exposure to blood borne illnesses such as HIV. Thanks to private funding, needle exchange programs are becoming more common, especially in large urban areas.

Where needle exchange programs aren't available, injection drug users must take steps to minimize exposure to blood borne illnesses. The equipment of drug use, commonly known as "works," includes needles, syringes, bowls, filters, spoons, water and citric acid. While using a new needle and syringe is preferable, properly cleaning the "works" prior to injecting drugs can help reduce the risk of HIV infection.

- Draw cold, clean water into the syringe and needle, and flush. Repeat two more times for a total of three.
- Draw household bleach into the syringe and needle. Let the bleach stand in the syringe for 30 seconds, then flush. Repeat this procedure two more times for a total of three.
- Draw cold, clean water into the syringe and needle, and flush. Repeat two more times for a total of three.

Keep in mind that cleaning your "works" in this manner will kill HIV; yet it does little to prevent the transmission of Hepatitis C, another epidemic fueled by needle sharing.

Positive Prevention

A common misconception is that HIV prevention stops once a person becomes HIV infected. Nothing could be further from the truth. Obviously, prevention techniques such as condoms must be used to prevent HIV exposure to those not infected. But what precautions need to be taken in relationships with two positive partners? Simply put, the same precautions that are taken in HIV negative couples. The concept of *positive prevention* refers to safer sex precautions taken in HIV positive couples to prevent *HIV reinfection.*

HIV REINFECTION

For many years, experts suspected that HIV-infected partners could reinfect one another. But until recently, the proof of reinfection was scare. With emerging data confirming what scientists have suspected for years, preventing HIV reinfection has become a new focus of prevention specialists around the country. HIV reinfection occurs when HIV-positive partners expose one another to their specific HIV virus. Because of natural changes or mutations that occur, HIV can vary slightly from person to person. When HIV infected people expose one another to their own specific HIV types, a mixing of two HIV types can occur, potentially resulting in one partner having multiple types of virus to treat.

HIV reinfection can complicate an already complicated illness. For example, person A has a type of HIV that is effectively treated by Drug #1. His partner, person B, has a type of HIV that is not treated effectively by Drug #1. If person A is reinfected by person B, there is a new HIV variant introduced to person A, one that is not treated effectively by Drug #1. The resulting mix of HIV types means person A must find a new drug to treat his HIV. Reinfection has made his old drug regimen ineffective, allowing his HIV to multiply and damage his immune system, which eventually will lead to infection and illness. Because of the potential harm caused by reinfection, barrier methods of safer sex, specifically latex condoms, must be used — just as if the couple were HIV negative.

HIV Testing Basics

Another important aspect of HIV prevention is testing. The Centers for Disease Control estimates that over 800,000 people in the United States are infected with HIV, but, incredibly, more than 200,000 of them are unaware they are infected. One only has to look to Africa to see the public health disaster that exists when people are not aware of their infection.

THE PRICE OF NOT KNOWING

Knowing one's status is paramount to staying healthy and slowing the HIV epidemic. What are the advantages of early diagnosis? What are the consequences of not knowing?

Early Intervention and Care

HIV testing and diagnosis allows for earlier access to medical care, which greatly improves the prognosis of people infected with HIV. Experts universally agree that early HIV medical care keeps a person healthier for a longer period of time. The availability of effective HIV medications allows the HIV specialist to treat the disease, thereby preserving the immune system and health of the infected individual. But to access care, a person needs to take that first step and get HIV tested.

HIV Prevention

Being unaware of HIV infection greatly impacts HIV prevention efforts. While the presence of an HIV infection is no guarantee, individuals have a greater incentive and are more likely to use safer sex methods if an infection is known to exist. With knowledge of an HIV infection, mothers who would otherwise choose to breast feed would bottle feed, thereby protecting their children from HIV exposure and infection. In the over-fifty population, many believe that condoms are used only to prevent pregnancy. Therefore, since becoming pregnant is not a concern in post-menopausal women over fifty, condoms are not used. Being aware of an HIV infection increases the probability that condoms will be used.

Knowing your HIV status is an important part of HIV prevention efforts. Knowing you are infected allows you to change behaviors that put you and others at risk. If positive, it allows you to get medical care sooner rather than later. Knowing your status answers the question "Can I infect others?" And if you are negative, being aware of that will relieve the anxiety and stress of not knowing.

HIV TESTING METHODS

Testing for HIV can be accomplished in many ways. Testing can be confidential or anonymous, free or for a fee, at home or in a testing facility, and by drawing blood from a vein or taking saliva from the mouth. Let's explore each of these testing options.

Confidential vs. Anonymous

For some, HIV testing can be a very threatening experience. Prejudices and stereotypes surrounding HIV are well known. There are people who avoid testing because they fear the social backlash of a positive test. Some even are fearful that the very test itself will label them, regardless of the result. For this reason, two methods of HIV testing exist: confidential and anonymous. Table 3 illustrates the differences.

- *Confidential*: These tests are usually done through commercial laboratories or medical practices. The person being tested provides his or her name, address, and other vital information prior to testing. The results of the test, positive or negative, are stored indefinitely according to name and are readily available to anyone permitted to access the medical records kept at the testing facility. While all medical practices and hospitals have a strict policy of confidentiality regarding medical information, there are no guarantees.

- *Anonymous*: This type of testing is done by community agencies, in-home test kits and free-standing testing facilities. No name is ever associated with the test, and no connection can be made between the person being tested and the random code assigned to him or her. Results are kept for a brief period, usually several weeks, and then destroyed. Anonymous testing provides the privacy and safety that people require in order to alleviate their fear of HIV testing.

TABLE 3

Confidential Testing

- Typically done through commercial labs, hospitals, or medical practices.
- There will be identifiers attached to the test and results (e.g., name, address, telephone, etc.).
- The results are stored indefinitely and are forever attached to the identifiers.
- Typically, these tests are done for a fee and may or may not be covered by medical insurance.
- Regulations try and assure confidentiality, but, unfortunately, there are no guarantees.
- Results are readily available to anyone permitted to view the facility's medical records.

Anonymous Testing

- Typically done in community agencies, free-standing testing and HIV facilities, and as part of home test kits.
- No name is ever associated with the test or the results.
- While unique identifiers (random numeric codes) are used, there is no way to connect test results to a specific person.
- Results are kept for a brief period of time and then destroyed.
- These tests are typically free of charge.

Free vs. Fee

HIV testing can be very expensive for those without financial means or medical insurance. The inability to pay deters people from being tested. To assure testing is readily accessible, two types are available.

- *For a Fee*: These tests are usually provided by medical practices, hospitals and laboratories. Coincidentally, these tests are usually confidential, as opposed to anonymous. Testing fees vary in amount but are paid for by most types of medical insurance.
- *Free*: As the name implies, these tests are free of charge. Most often these tests are provided by HIV testing organizations and are usually anony-

mous. Government-funded testing programs also provide free tests through state and local agencies, and county health departments.

Home vs. Community Testing

The majority of tests, both confidential and anonymous, are done in the community in testing agencies, medical practices, laboratories, and hospitals. But, as mentioned earlier, HIV testing can be a very scary and threatening experience to many people. In an effort to engage those people reluctant to be tested because of anxiety and fear, the FDA has approved home testing as an alternative to community testing.

- *Home Testing*: Home test kits are available without a prescription at local pharmacies. Saliva is collected by swabbing the inside of the cheek. The swab is packaged according to instructions provided as part of the kit and mailed to a testing laboratory. Much like anonymous testing, a random code is assigned to each kit. With this code, the user can retrieve test results by telephone. While the home test kit does provide the privacy people want, test accuracy has come into question. Some manufacturers' kits are more reliable than others, creating an air of uncertainty surrounding home tests. Any positive result or a negative result in the presence of significant HIV risk factors should be confirmed by a test provided by a community agency or lab.

- *Community Testing*: Community testing is done in testing agencies, hospitals, laboratories, and medical practices. Community agencies usually use the cheek swab method similar to those used in home test kits. Laboratories, hospitals, and medical practices, on the other hand, use blood samples drawn from a vein. Unlike home test kits, community testing is considered more reliable and accurate by the person being tested, as well as by the medical community. Depending on the testing site, community testing can be free and anonymous, or for a fee and confidential.

HOW DO HIV TESTS WORK?

To understand HIV testing, you first must understand what occurs in the body when HIV enters the blood stream. The *immune system* is the body's defense against foreign organisms and infectious agents, such as HIV. The immune system senses a foreign invader and produces substances known as *antibodies* that attempt to fight off the infectious agent. Antibodies are specific to the organism they are fighting. For instance, the body produces hepatitis B antibodies to fight off hepatitis B, and flu antibodies to fight off the flu. Likewise, when your body is exposed to HIV, antibodies are produced that are specific to HIV. It's these specific HIV antibodies that are detected by HIV tests. When HIV enters the blood stream, HIV antibodies are produced, which are then detected by HIV testing. If antibodies are detected, the HIV test is positive and the person is said to be HIV-infected.

There are three types of HIV antibody tests used to detect HIV infection.

- *ELISA*: The ELISA test is actually a laboratory technique used to detect HIV antibodies. It is most often used on blood, but can be used to test saliva (as in the cheek swab tests) and urine. The ELISA is the first testing technique used on a blood sample because it's very sensitive and rarely provides "false negative" results (negative results in the presence of HIV antibodies). "False positive" results, or positive test results in the absence of HIV antibodies, are much more common. Because of this, ELISA testing alone can't diagnose an HIV infection. If the ELISA test results are negative, the testing process ends and the person is considered not to be HIV-infected at that time. If the ELISA test is positive, the testing process moves to the next step, the Western Blot Assay.

- *Western Blot Assay (WB)*: The Western Blot Assay is another technique that is only used after the ELISA test is positive. Because of the very rare incidence of "false positive" results, this test is used to confirm the results of the ELISA. The test looks for the presence of HIV *protein bands* in the blood being tested. Proteins are organic compounds that make up living organisms. HIV is made up of HIV proteins. If three or more of these HIV protein bands are detected, the sample is said to be Western Blot positive, confirming the positive ELISA. While the ELISA has two possible results, "positive" or "negative," the Western Blot has three:

  - *Positive*: Three or more proteins are present, confirming the sample as being HIV-infected.
  - *Negative*: No HIV protein bands are present, and the sample is considered not to be HIV-infected.
  - *Indeterminant*: One or two protein bands are present. This result is neither positive nor negative. If a sample is indeterminant, and if the person being tested has HIV risk factors or has a known HIV exposure, another test should be performed in six to twelve weeks.

- *Indirect Immunofluorescence Assay (IFA)*: The IFA testing method is seldom used but acts as a confirmatory test, much like the Western Blot. Faster than a Western Blot, labs sometimes use the IFA when the speed in which results are obtained is an issue.

WHEN NEGATIVE ISN'T NEGATIVE

At first glance, a negative Western Blot test means that there is no HIV infection. A majority of the time this is true, but there is a circumstance when the ELISA and Western Blot tests can be negative, yet the person can still be HIV-infected. How is that possible?

The body has a built-in defense mechanism that detects infectious organisms and produces specific antibodies that help fight the organism. If HIV antibodies are present, the person is HIV positive; if not, they are HIV negative. The problem is that the body needs time to manufacture these HIV antibodies, meaning the test has some degree of inaccuracy.

There is a "window of time" between when HIV enters the blood stream and when enough HIV antibodies have been produced by the body to be detected by HIV tests. It's during this "window" that a person will have a negative HIV test despite having HIV in their blood. Simply put, in this case, negative doesn't necessarily mean negative. More importantly, despite having a negative test, the person is infectious and can transmit HIV to other people.

In order for a test to be considered accurate, the body must be given ample time to produce antibodies in quantities great enough to be detected by HIV testing. This is accomplished by performing a series of HIV tests—at six weeks, three months and finally six months after a potential exposure. If after the six month test there are still no HIV antibodies detected, a person can feel confident that he or she is not HIV-infected.

So what if the test is positive? What happens next? Where do we go from here?

3

HIV 101 ... The Basics

Understanding HIV and AIDS starts with understanding the basics. HIV 101, as it is called, is an essential first step to building the strong foundation needed to live with the disease. Someone once said that the best place to start is the beginning. It all begins with a virus. Before we can understand HIV, we must first understand viruses and why they need us to survive.

What Is a Virus?

As the name implies, Human Immunodeficiency Virus (HIV) is a virus. But what exactly is a virus? By definition, a virus is a microscopic living organism that makes copies of itself by using genetic material from the cells of a living host. Specifically, there are two types of genetic material needed for viruses to replicate: *Ribonucleic Acid (RNA)* and *Deoxyribonucleic Acid (DNA)*. Big words, but what do they mean?

RNA is a single strand protein that is one of the building blocks of living organisms. The role of RNA is to transport genetic information to the site where new proteins are being manufactured. *DNA* is a double strand protein building block that contains the genetic information needed during the manufacture of new proteins. It's that genetic information that makes a virus a virus, a monkey a monkey, or a human a human. Through chemical reactions, DNA is changed to RNA. The RNA then transports the genetic code of the DNA to the sites of protein manufacturing. On a car assembly line, parts for the car must be brought to the line so they can be assembled. RNA brings the genetic parts to the protein assembly line.

In most living organisms, including viruses, DNA is converted to RNA in the process of making more viral copies. HIV, on the other hand, is a *retrovirus,* meaning they convert RNA to DNA in order to make more copies. A key point to remember is that virus and retrovirus, both types, need genetic material from a living host in order to survive and multiply. In the case of HIV, we

34

are the living host and our cellular RNA is changed into viral DNA in order to make more HIV copies.

The HIV Life Cycle

What happens after HIV enters the blood stream? How does HIV make copies of itself? The HIV life cycle is comprised of many steps, each with a very specific and important role in the replication of HIV.

INTRODUCTION OF HIV INTO THE BODY

Before HIV can replicate, it must enter the body. As we learned earlier, exposure to infected bodily fluids during sexual contact or by sharing needles are the primary means by which HIV enters the body. While less common, HIV can also enter the body during pregnancy, child birth or by ingesting HIV-infected breast milk.

VIRAL ATTACHMENT

Once in the body, HIV needs a *host cell* in order to replicate. In the case of HIV, the host is a specialized cell from the immune system known as the *T-cell* or *CD4 cell*. Once in the bloodstream, HIV seeks out and attaches to the CD4 cell in a "lock and key" system. Proteins on the surface of HIV attach to complimentary proteins on the CD4 cell much the way a key fits into a lock. Once attached to the CD4 cell, HIV can move on to the next step in the life cycle.

VIRAL FUSION

Once attached to the cell, HIV injects proteins of its own into the cellular fluids (cytoplasm) of the CD4 cell. This causes a *fusion* or joining of the host cell membrane to the outer envelope of HIV. As part of this fusing, a fusion pore develops, creating a "tunnel" between the virus and the CD4 cell. It's through this "tunnel" that the HIV genetic material enters the healthy CD4 cell.

THE UNCOATING

In order for HIV to use its genetic material (RNA) for reproduction, the protective coating surrounding the RNA strand must be dissolved. Not much is known about this step, but one thing is certain — without this step, conversion of HIV RNA to DNA can't take place, and replication is halted.

REVERSE TRANSCRIPTION

Once in the cell, the single-stranded HIV RNA must be converted to double-stranded DNA. This takes place with the help of the enzyme *reverse transcriptase.* Reverse transcriptase uses proteins from the CD4 cell to help change the HIV RNA to HIV DNA. Reverse transcriptase allows genetic information to flow in the opposite direction (RNA to DNA), as opposed to the normal direction (DNA to RNA). The resulting DNA contains the viral genetic information needed for HIV replication to continue to the next step.

INTEGRATION

To use the cell during replication, HIV must *integrate* or insert its newly formed DNA into the CD4 cell's *nucleus.* The nucleus is considered the brain of the cell, containing all of the RNA and DNA of that cell. Integration is accomplished with the help of an *enzyme* called *retroviral integrase.* Enzymes are special proteins that start or help a chemical reaction to occur. Retroviral integrase fuels the chemical reaction that inserts the viral DNA into the CD4 cell.

VIRAL LATENCY

Webster's Dictionary defines *latency* as an incubation period or a period of waiting. HIV must wait for additional proteins to be manufactured before replication can be completed. This period of waiting is known as viral latency.

FINAL ASSEMBLY

Once the viral proteins are manufactured, they must be cut in pieces and assembled into new HIV particles. This *cleavage* or cutting is accomplished with the help of another protein enzyme called *protease.* The enzyme cuts the proteins into smaller pieces, allowing those pieces to reassemble into new HIV particles.

BUDDING

Budding is the final step in the HIV life cycle. The newly formed HIV, complete with viral genetic material and a new outer coat made from the cell membrane of the host CD4 cell, "pinches off" of the host cell and enters the body's circulation. After a period of maturation — an HIV "growing up," so to speak — the newly formed HIV is ready to attach to another CD4 cell and start the process all over again. The process of HIV replication destroys the host CD4 cells while producing hundreds of thousands of active HIV copies. What effect does this have on the human body?

The Immune System

The body's defense against parasites, bacteria, viruses and other sources of infection is the *immune system.* The immune system is composed of specialized cells, organs, and a circulatory system all working together to detect foreign substances and organisms that can cause infection. Once an infectious agent is detected, an *immune response* is initiated that protects the body by killing the foreign invader. For example, when a cold virus enters the body, the immune system detects the virus and produces a response that fights the cold. While the virus is able to produce cold symptoms, the immune system limits the severity and duration of those symptoms.

How Does the Immune System Work?

Foreign organisms that enter the body are called *antigens*. Once in the body, these antigens are detected by the immune system, triggering the production of antibodies that help fight off the infectious agent. Antibodies attach to the antigen in a manner very similar to the lock and key method that HIV uses to attach to the CD4 cell. Antibodies are specific to the antigen they attach to—the way a key is specific to the lock it opens. Once attached, the antibody "tags" the antigen, allowing other cells of the immune system to recognize and destroy it before it causes illness or disease.

Once antibodies are produced, they remain in the body, standing guard in case the antigen that triggered their production enters the body some other time. For instance, when the chickenpox virus enters the body, our immune system produces antibodies that help rid the body of the virus. Once the virus has been eliminated, the antibody remains, providing us with *immunity*, or protection, from future exposures to chickenpox. Because of this, once you've had chickenpox, you have lifelong protection, meaning you will not get chickenpox again even if you are exposed.

What Occurs After HIV Enters the Body

Remember from the discussion about the HIV life cycle that the virus needs our genetic material to make more viral copies. The virus gets the genetic material it needs by attaching and fusing to CD4 cells. Specifically, HIV attaches to highly specialized cells in our immune system called T-cells or CD4 cells. When a foreign antigen is detected, CD4 cells instruct other immune system cells to start making antibodies. CD4 cells also activate specialized cells that attack and destroy host cells that have been infected by the foreign antigen. It's obvious that CD4 cells play a very important role in the immune response.

Unfortunately, the process of HIV replication destroys the CD4 cell. As HIV attaches to more and more CD4 cells, the number of functioning CD4 cells decreases. Imagine an army of CD4 soldiers guarding the body from enemy viruses—in this case, HIV. The enemy sneaks into the body, catching the soldiers off guard. HIV attacks the soldiers, destroying them one by one. Eventually, so many soldiers are destroyed that those remaining are unable to protect the body from the enemy. As the example illustrates, HIV replication damages so many CD4 cells that the immune system becomes weak and unable to protect the body from foreign antigens.

Does HIV Make You Sick?

Over twenty years ago when the epidemic started, people died shortly after being diagnosed with AIDS. Today that's no longer true; but after being infected, people do get sick from time to time. Is it HIV that makes us sick? Indirectly, the answer is yes, but HIV itself doesn't cause illness or infection. If that's the case, why do people get sick after being infected with HIV? Why did people die twenty years ago?

During the replication process, HIV destroys CD4 cells, which, over time, weakens our immune system. By fighting off infections and other illnesses, a strong immune system keeps us healthy. A weak immune system means a body at risk for infections caused by foreign antigens. Eventually the body is unable to fight off any infectious agent, resulting in serious illness and, in some cases, death. Keep in mind that this is the natural course of an HIV infection without medical intervention. Medications alter this scenario significantly. To better understand the process, let's look at it step by step.

Step 1: HIV enters the blood stream and begins to replicate, using CD4 cells as the source of genetic material.

Step 2: As more copies of HIV are made, more and more CD4 cells are destroyed, gradually weakening the immune system.

Step 3: As HIV replication continues, the immune system eventually becomes unable to fight off infection.

Step 4: With little or no functioning immune system, infectious organisms find minimal resistance when they enter the body. Soon, infection is common, eventually leading to serious illness and death.

Infectious organisms take advantage of weak immune systems, seizing the opportunity to cause sickness. It's the *opportunistic infections* that make people sick, not HIV.

HIV vs. AIDS

The mainstream media, lay people, and even some health care providers use the terms HIV and AIDS interchangeably. For many, HIV and AIDS are one in the same. Actually, they're not the same at all.

Acquired Immune Deficiency Syndrome, or AIDS for short, is actually the name given to the most serious opportunistic infections that strike when the immune system is at its weakest. These AIDS-defining illnesses include:

- Candidiasis of bronchi, trachea, or lungs
- Candidiasis, esophageal
- Cervical cancer, invasive
- Coccidioidomycosis, disseminated or extrapulmonary
- Cryptococcosis, extrapulmonary
- Cryptosporidiosis, chronic intestinal (greater than 1 month's duration)
- Cytomegalovirus disease (other than liver, spleen, or nodes)
- Cytomegalovirus retinitis (with loss of vision)
- Encephalopathy, HIV-related
- Herpes simplex: chronic ulcer(s) (greater than 1 month's duration); or bronchitis, pneumonitis, or esophagitis
- Histoplasmosis, disseminated or extrapulmonary
- Isosporiasis, chronic intestinal (greater than 1 month's duration)
- Kaposi's sarcoma (KS)
- Lymphoma, Burkitt's (or equivalent term)
- Lymphoma, immunoblastic (or equivalent term)
- Lymphoma, primary, of brain
- Mycobacterium avium complex or M. kansasii, disseminated or extrapulmonary
- Mycobacterium tuberculosis, any site (pulmonary or extrapulmonary)
- Mycobacterium, other species or unidentified species, disseminated or extrapulmonary
- Pneumocystis carinii pneumonia (PCP)
- Pneumonia, recurrent
- Progressive multifocal leukoencephalopathy (PML)
- Salmonella septicemia, recurrent
- Toxoplasmosis of brain
- Wasting syndrome due to HIV

It's not important to remember the complex medical names of all the AIDS-defining illnesses. Just remember that if a person has ever been diagnosed with one of them, he or she is said to have AIDS. AIDS is a result of immune system damage, and HIV causes that damage. As you can see, HIV and AIDS are definitely connected, but they are certainly not the same thing.

The Significance of an AIDS Diagnosis

Being diagnosed with one of the AIDS-defining opportunistic infections is not the only way to be classified as having AIDS. An AIDS diagnosis can also be made according to the total CD4 count. The number of CD4 cells is measured by a simple blood test. The normal value ranges between 500 and 1,500 CD4 cells per cubic milliliter of blood. When the CD4 level falls below 200 CD4 cells per cubic milliliter of blood, the person is said to have AIDS.

What is the significance of an AIDS diagnosis? When the epidemic emerged twenty years ago, an AIDS diagnosis signaled that the end of life was near. Prior to the development of an HIV test, people were diagnosed after they exhibited symptoms of an AIDS-defining infection. By the time symptoms of infection appeared, the disease was in an advanced stage, already having done irreparable damage to the immune system. Most often peopled died within months of an AIDS diagnosis. Obviously, twenty years ago, being diagnosed with AIDS was very significant.

Since the development of the HIV test, people are diagnosed much earlier in the course of the disease. The advent of HIV medications has delayed the progression to AIDS for many years. Even after an AIDS diagnosis is made, medications keep people healthy and alive for a very long time. AIDS is no longer the death sentence it was two decades ago and is nowhere near as significant today as it was then.

Tracking the epidemic is an important part of HIV prevention and care. Federal funds are allocated based on the epidemic patterns among populations and geographic areas. At the beginning of the epidemic, the only way to track the epidemic was to count the number of AIDS cases. Because people were diagnosed only after they acquired AIDS-defining infections, the number of AIDS cases was an accurate representation of the number of HIV-infected people.

Today, counting the number of AIDS cases is not an accurate method of tracking the epidemic. HIV testing makes it possible to diagnose people long before they have AIDS-defining infections. Counting only AIDS cases would be inaccurate because the method omits a large number of people with HIV that have yet to progress to AIDS, and may not for several years. While many attach great significance to an AIDS diagnosis, the fact is that AIDS is in many ways an outdated classification that has outlived its usefulness.

The Natural Course of HIV

Without medications or medical intervention, HIV is free to follow its natural course and, in the process, destroy the immune system. Soon after infection, HIV begins replicating at a very rapid pace, damaging CD4 cells along the way. Early in infection, the amount of circulating virus is very high, and the number of functioning CD4 cells declines drastically. Simply put, HIV has caught the immune system off guard. Three to six weeks after being infected, many people experience a flu-like illness known as acute HIV infection. Symptoms include fever, diarrhea, rash, fatigue, malaise, and weight loss. Quite often, the symptoms are attributed to the flu or some other viral illness. Because the body has not had ample time to develop antibodies, an HIV test can be negative, despite the presence of HIV in the blood. Many times, the opportunity of early diagnosis is missed because of the negative HIV test and symptoms that could be attributed to other illnesses.

About six weeks after infection, most people will have developed enough HIV antibodies to be detected by the HIV test. Once antibodies are formed, the body begins to fight the new infection. The symptoms of the acute infection resolve and the person begins to feel much better, confirming their mistaken belief that what they experienced was nothing more than a typical viral illness.

As the body begins to realize what is happening, the remaining healthy CD4 cells begin to fight HIV. About six months into the infection the immune system is successful in stabilizing the number of circulating HIV at a level known as the viral load *set point*. The set point varies from person to person and can be a predictor of how fast HIV will progress to AIDS in the future.

Once the set point is reached, the virus begins a chronic phase during which the body's immune system is able to suppress viral replication enough to maintain the strength of the immune system. The duration of this chronic phase can vary greatly from person to person, ranging from a year to ten years or more. During this time, the infected person feels well and has few, if any, symptoms. Because a stable CD4 count can be maintained, the immune system is able to protect the body from opportunistic infections, and the person's overall health remains good.

Years after the initial infection, HIV replication continues, slowly chipping away at the number of healthy CD4 cells. Eventually, so many CD4 cells are destroyed by HIV that the immune system is significantly weakened and the body becomes at risk for opportunistic infections. Remember the normal CD4 count ranges from 500 to 1500 cells per cubic milliliter of blood. When the level falls below 200 cells per cubic milliliter of blood the person is at significant risk for the most serious opportunistic infections, and is diagnosed as having AIDS.

Still, HIV replication continues, and opportunistic infections become more common as the number of functioning CD4 cells continue to decline. Once the level falls below 100 CD4 cells per cubic milliliter of blood, HIV becomes stronger than the immune system, and the most serious, potentially fatal opportunistic infections become commonplace. Without some sort of medical intervention, the body will soon be unable to fight any infection, eventually leading to the person's death.

Typically, people live on average about 10 to 15 years without any type of treatment. Some people with more aggressive strains of HIV survive as little as a couple of years, while others with less aggressive strains of HIV can live twenty or more years.

The Long Term Non-Progressor

The natural progression of HIV infection slowly destroys the immune system, lowering the CD4 count over the course of several years. Some people infected with HIV are *long term non-progressor,* maintaining stable CD4 counts for ten years or more without any medical intervention or HIV medications. Research is being conducted to determine why some people progress slower than others. Understanding long term non-progressors could result in new and better HIV treatments that may extend the lives of HIV-infected people even further.

Now that we understand the basics of HIV and AIDS, the discussion turns to those first days and weeks after diagnosis. If the HIV test result is positive, what comes next?

4

The Test Is Positive ...
Now What?

Many people are reluctant to be HIV tested because they're afraid of what it would do to their lives if they were indeed HIV positive. Being diagnosed with any chronic and potentially fatal disease is frightening, but a diagnosis of HIV gives a new meaning to the word fear. So what if the unthinkable does occur? What if that HIV test is positive? The first few days and weeks can be the most important and the most difficult. Making the right choices from the beginning can mean the difference between you taking control of your disease or your disease taking control of you.

Pre- and Post-Test Counseling

Getting HIV tested entails a lot more than just holding out your arm and having blood drawn. HIV testing is more than just finding out if you are positive or negative. It's an opportunity to educate and an opportunity to learn. Testing policy and procedure varies from state to state. About twenty percent of states require pre-test and/or post-test counseling, with many being very specific regarding what HIV counseling must include. The United States Department of Health and Human Services recommends that counseling include an explanation of the HIV test itself; basic HIV and AIDS information; methods to diminish the risk of spreading HIV from person to person; the importance of test confidentiality; the possible social impact of being HIV tested; and, finally, who needs to be made aware of positive results. Post-test counseling provides an opportunity for medical and psychosocial referrals in the event of a positive test. If the test is negative, post-test counseling provides an opportunity to share information that will diminish the risk of HIV exposure.

What Happens During Pre-Test Counseling?

Prior to getting your HIV test, you will meet with a specially trained and certified HIV test counselor. Test counselors will ask questions about your medical history and any behaviors that may put you at risk for HIV exposure, such as unprotected sex, trading sex for drugs, or having sex with known HIV positive people. The counselor will also ask about any history of recreational drug use or sharing needles while injecting drugs. The purpose of these intimate questions is to assess your HIV risk and to counsel you on ways to reduce or avoid risky behaviors in the future.

As part of your pre-test counseling, the HIV counselor will explain the basics of HIV and AIDS, including transmission routes, methods of safer sex and ways to reduce your risk of infection. He or she will discuss the social impact HIV testing has on the person being tested. Finally, you will have an opportunity to ask questions of the test counselor. When all your questions have been answered, the counselor will make certain you are still interested in being tested. If so, you will sign a consent form and take the test.

What Happens During Post-Test Counseling?

Depending on the type of HIV test you have and where you have it, your test results will be ready anywhere from ten minutes to several days. Your test counselor will have you come into the test center for your results. Test results, either negative or positive, will never be given over the telephone. Receiving your results is more than just learning if you're positive or negative. If your test is negative, your counselor will again discuss safer sex methods, ways to reduce your risk of HIV exposure, and the importance of not sharing needles. Your counselor will also discuss the importance of repeating your test several weeks later to confirm your negative results. Finally, depending on the testing site, condoms are available in order to encourage their use during each and every sexual encounter.

Receiving positive test results is a very stressful and emotional event. Shock, fear, anger, and disbelief are all common emotions after learning you are HIV-infected. Your test counselor is specially trained to help deal with the onslaught of emotions and the adjustments that need to be made after receiving your positive results. The counselor will assist with medical referrals and, if needed, mental health referrals. Finally, the counselor will explain who you must tell, and help you decide who, if anyone, you want to tell about your positive test results.

TABLE 4

Pre-Test Counseling
- The purpose of pre-test counseling is to assess HIV risk.
- Trained and certified test counselors will take a medical and sexual history.
- Sexual history will include the number of partners; questions regarding trading sex for drugs; and any history of having sex with anonymous partners.
- The counselor will ask about any history of recreational drug use or sharing needles.
- Part of your pre-test counseling is an explanation of basic HIV/AIDS information.
- Some pre-test counseling involves a discussion of the social impact of HIV and being tested.
- Finally, you will be given the option of being tested now that you have all the information.

Post-Test Counseling
- Keep in mind, test results, either positive or negative, will never be given by telephone.
- If your test is negative, your counselor will discuss safer sex methods and ways to reduce your HIV risk.
- The counselor will discuss ways to decrease your risk of HIV when injecting drugs, including offering to refer you to substance abuse treatment.
- The counselor will instruct you on the importance of being retested several weeks later to confirm the results.
- If your results are positive, your counselor will assist with medical referrals, mental health referrals, and will help with the initial shock of a positive diagnosis.
- Often, condoms will be available to take with you after post-test counseling.

A Positive Test ... Taking the First Steps

Being diagnosed with HIV can be an incredible shock, filling a person with fear, desperation, and confusion. The initial reaction may be to throw in the towel, to give up and let the disease take control. Like any medical diagnosis, learning you are HIV-infected is not the news anyone wants to hear. Every person will handle the news differently. For many, the initial reaction may be to give up and let HIV take control. Others choose to cope by using alcohol or drugs. Still others will deny they have any illness at all.

Initially, most people will feel helpless, but the truth is it's possible to take control of your life while living with HIV. To do so requires preparation, determination, and the will to move forward. There are several things that must be done in order to move forward with an HIV diagnosis. They include:

- deciding whether to tell, and who to tell, about your diagnosis;
- take control of your life; and
- finding a qualified HIV specialist willing to work with you.

Each is an essential step when preparing for a life with HIV. Let's look at each a little closer.

Who Do You Tell About Your HIV?

As is true with all medical information, HIV test results are strictly confidential. For the most part, it's the individual's decision who to tell, if anyone, about their HIV status. However, there are circumstances that require HIV-infected people to disclose their HIV status.

You Must Disclose

HIV disclosure laws vary from state to state. Most require that a person make their HIV status known to any potential sexual partner prior to sexual contact or intimacy. Knowingly exposing a sexual partner to HIV without their knowledge is, in most cases, a criminal act, punishable as a felony.

Disclosure Is Recommended

While it's not required, it is recommended that you disclose your HIV status to other doctors, dentists, and medical providers that care for you. The purpose of disclosure is not to protect your medical providers from potential HIV infection. Medical professionals employ the same universal precautions for all patients, regardless of their HIV status. The fact is that disclosing your HIV status benefits you. All medical providers need a complete picture of your health and medical history to care for you properly. Having HIV can impact the way other conditions are treated and how certain symptoms are interpreted. Most experts agree that disclosing your HIV status to all of your health care providers is a good idea.

The Choice Is Yours

Disclosing your HIV status to anyone else other than those people in the previous examples is strictly your decision. Before disclosing, ask yourself why you are doing so and what will be gained. For instance, telling your family of your diagnosis may provide you with a support system to help you cope with your new diagnosis. On the other hand, disclosing your status to coworkers or casual acquaintances may not benefit you at all. Keep in mind that disclosing your status is not something to take lightly and should be thought out carefully before doing so.

TABLE 5

Mandatory Disclosure
- Past sexual partners.
- Potential sexual partners prior to any sexual contact.

Recommended Disclosure
- Doctors, dentists, and any medical professionals that will be caring for you.

The Choice is Yours
- Friends, family, acquaintances, and employers.

How to Disclose Your HIV Status

Telling someone you have HIV, be it a loved one or your best friend, can be one of the hardest things you will ever have to do. You may feel awkward, afraid, or embarrassed. The person you are telling will certainly react in any number of ways. Some may be angry, others will be sad. Some will be frightened and still others won't know exactly how they feel. While the task of disclosure is a difficult one, there are steps you can take to prepare for the task.

- Learn as much as you can about HIV. Knowledge is power. Having an understanding of HIV and AIDS will allow you to answer questions and ease the fears of the person you are telling.
- Know why you want to tell the people you are telling. What do you want from them? Are they at risk for infection? Have you unknowingly exposed them to your HIV? Will they be a source of support? Have an idea why you are disclosing before you disclose.
- Anticipate their reaction. What's the best you can hope for? What's the worst you will have to deal with? Often, the person you tell will experience emotions much like you did when you were told of the diagnosis. Be prepared for a variety of emotions ranging from anger to fear. Ironically, you may have to be their support before they can be yours.
- To promote an understanding of HIV and AIDS, have educational materials on hand to help answer questions that may arise.
- If you have someone who already knows your status, bring them along for support, both for you and the person you are telling. Along with that person, come up with a disclosure plan. While it may not always be appropriate to bring along another person, a support person can help come up with a plan of action prior to disclosure, making the process much less stressful.
- Be prepared for any reaction and allow the person you are telling to express their emotions freely. Often the person being told will need as much support as the person who is disclosing their HIV status. Remember, you can't control the fears and feelings of others, and it may take time for the person to adjust to and accept what you have told them.
- Be patient. It may take some time for those you tell to process the information and be supportive of you. Everyone deals with difficult news in their own way and in their own time.

Partner Notification

One type of HIV disclosure is partner notification. HIV can remain undiagnosed for several years. During that time an HIV infected person can unknowingly expose their sexual partners to the virus. Because early diagnosis is so important, an infected person must notify their past sexual partners that they may have been exposed to HIV. This allows those people potentially exposed to get HIV tested and into medical care if they are found to be HIV-infected. Partner notification also provides a means by which HIV exposure between sexual partners can be reduced, which in turn will slow the spread of HIV. There are three ways to notify a partner.

NOTIFICATION BY THE INFECTED PERSON

Partner notification can be done by the HIV-infected person. Hearing about a potential exposure can sometimes be easier if the news is delivered by a partner, loved one or friend. However, it can also be a very awkward encounter. Many infected people would rather not be the one to pass on such troubling news. Doctors, counselors or social workers can offer support to those people who wish to notify their partners themselves.

NOTIFICATION BY THE LOCAL HEALTH DEPARTMENT

In most states, new HIV infections are reported to the local health department. Even in circumstances where little is known about past sexual encounters, the health department can assist in partner notification. For instance, people meeting for anonymous sexual encounters may know little about one another. The local health department can take any little bit of information, such as a first name or where the sexual encounter took place, and track down the person or persons potentially exposed.

The involvement of local health departments is not limited to anonymous encounters. Health department staff can assist in notifying known partners as well. Despite their diligence in finding and notifying sexual partners, they take great care not to compromise the confidentiality of the HIV-infected person. Notification is vague, making the person aware that they may have been in contact with someone HIV-infected without giving specifics about the person who exposed them.

NOTIFICATION BY THE PHYSICIAN

Physicians caring for newly diagnosed HIV-infected people can do partner notification as well. In fact, many states require physicians to perform partner notification, or, at the very least, make sure the infected person or the health department notifies those people exposed. Most times physicians have neither the resources nor the time to do a thorough and complete partner notification. Usually the task is delegated to social workers, nurses, the HIV-infected person or the local health department. Regardless of who does the notification, it's the physician's responsibility to make certain it's documented.

Take Control

Regardless of your personality, an HIV diagnosis can wreak havoc with your level of confidence. If you normally took control of situations before you were diagnosed, then you can take control now that you're HIV-infected. If taking charge came easy to you before, with hard work, support and time, it should again.

On the other hand, if you were one to let things happen around you or take a passive approach to life, needing to "step up" and take control may be intimidating. The tendency would be to sit back and let others take control of your health care. Taking a passive approach to your disease will shut you out of the process. Once you turn control over to others, it's very difficult to get it back. Without taking control, you become an outsider in your own health care. Taking control from the start assures that you will be included in every aspect of your health care. Arguably, taking control and being empowered is the key to staying healthy.

Fortunately, being able to take control of your life is something that can be learned. It requires very hard work and determination. At times the urge will be to quit and assume a passive role. Pushing forward, despite these urges, will help you move forward after your diagnosis. In order to move forward and take control of your life and disease, there are a few things you must learn first.

YOU ARE NUMBER ONE

Now that you have been diagnosed with HIV, your health and quality of life must become the most important thing in your life. Depending on your personality, this may be difficult for you. You may feel guilty or selfish, or have mixed feelings about putting your health first. If your relationship is one where your partner is in control, he or she may have trouble with you taking the lead in some aspects of life. It will take time for them to adjust to the "new you." Resist the tendency to revert back to the "old you." The work you and your partner will invest is worth it. Your health and well-being is much too important to leave in the hands of others.

Putting yourself first doesn't mean becoming isolated or abandoning your responsibilities. It does mean that it's okay and necessary to sometimes say "no." It's necessary to make your needs known to your doctor and the people around you. Learning to say no and expressing your needs is simply becoming empowered.

Women living with HIV tend to abandon their own needs in order to care for their family and children. When a woman takes care of herself, she is doing something good for her family as well. Doing what is needed to stay healthy allows a woman to care for others and teaches her children an important lesson — how to love yourself.

Finally, taking control also means resisting the temptation to think of yourself as "helpless" or as a "victim." Don't identify yourself or allow others to identify you by your diagnosis. You are not an "AIDS patient"; you are a person with a disease. That fact can never diminish the person you are or the respect you deserve. If you feel someone is treating you in a disrespectful manner, tell them.

BELIEVE IN YOURSELF

Nobody knows what's best for you except you. Who better to understand how you're feeling physically and emotionally than yourself. If you feel something is not right, even if you don't know why, then it's probably not. Know your body and trust your instincts. Survival is a very strong instinct that you should not ignore.

Chronic illness makes life more difficult but certainly not impossible. There needs to be adjustments and changes in your routine, and it will be a lot of work. But believe in yourself. Believe that you can make those adjustments and that you are up to the task; after all, your health hangs in the balance.

GIVE YOURSELF SOME TIME

Take a deep breath. You don't have to rush into any rash decisions now that you have HIV. Making decisions that impact your health and your life can't be made on a whim. Make sure you give yourself all the time you need. Decisions should be made according to *your* time frame, not that of the doctor, the nurse or anyone else. Have realistic expectations of yourself. Don't try to do too much too soon, and don't expect too much of yourself at the beginning. Change takes time, so make sure to leave yourself plenty.

TABLE 6. TAKE CONTROL OF YOUR LIFE

You are Number 1
- Your health and quality of life must become your highest priority.
- Feeling guilty or selfish, or having mixed feelings is common.
- Your partner or spouse may have trouble adjusting to you "taking the lead."
- If being the priority is new to you, resist reverting back to the "old you."
- Being first doesn't mean you need to isolate yourself.
- It is ok and sometimes necessary to say "no."
- It is necessary to make your wishes and needs known to your doctor.
- Women must not abandon their own needs for the needs of their children and family.

Believe in Yourself
- Nobody knows how you feel emotionally or physically better than you.
- If you feel something is not right, then it probably is not right, even if you don't know why.
- The survival instinct is very strong and should not be ignored ... in other words, trust your instincts.
- Difficult adjustments in your life will have to be made, but believe in yourself ... YOU CAN DO IT!
- You are up to the task.

Give Yourself Some Time
• Take a deep breath ... you have time to make the right choices.
• Do not rush into any rash decisions regarding your medical care or to whom you disclose your diagnosis.
• Decisions should be made on *your* timeframe, not your doctor's.
• Have realistic expectations ... don't try to do too much too soon.
• Change takes time, so leave yourself plenty.

Choosing a Doctor That's Right for You

The most important decision you will make in those first few days after learning you have HIV is choosing a doctor to take care of you. It's a decision that will impact your health as well as your quality of life for many years. Obviously it's not a decision you should take lightly. Take a systematic approach to finding the right doctor for you. Here are several things you should consider when choosing your doctor.

• *Find a Doctor:* To find a doctor you have to know where to look. In large urban areas, large medical centers or university-based hospitals are a good place to start. In urban areas hard hit by HIV, free-standing medical practices or clinics are a good source of quality HIV care. In rural areas it may be necessary to travel several miles to the nearest large city to get your HIV care. To minimize travel, a local family physician can be retained for illnesses and issues not related to HIV; but to care for your HIV, it's best to see an HIV specialist, even if it means some travel. If your search for an HIV specialist comes up empty, you can call the National AIDS Hotline at 1-800-342-2437. By providing your zip code, the hotline allows you to search for an HIV specialist wherever you live.

• *Find an HIV Specialist:* HIV is a very complex disease requiring expertise in HIV and infectious disease to be properly managed. HIV specialists are infectious disease doctors that further specialize in the treatment of patients with HIV and AIDS. However, being an infectious disease specialist is not enough. Experts recommend that people living with HIV should only trust their care to a doctor who treats at least fifty HIV-infected people per year. HIV is so complex, and treatment guidelines change so often, that doctors need to devote their full-time attention to HIV medicine. The doctor you choose should keep up to date on the most current advances in HIV medicine by attending continuing education conferences, and through extensive journal review. The importance of choosing an HIV specialist to manage your care can't be stressed enough.

• *Choose a Full Service Medical Practice:* HIV and AIDS affect the whole person, physically as well as emotionally. For that reason it is important to choose a doctor whose clinic offers more than just medical care. Does the clinic employ social workers, nutritionists, and nurses who specialize in HIV? Does the practice have access to specialty care such as ophthalmology, gynecology, substance abuse treatment and psychiatry? People living with HIV need more than just medical care. Choose a doctor that treats the entire person.

- *Choose a Doctor That Understands the Special Needs of HIV-Infected Women:* Women living with HIV have special needs that must be addressed by their doctor. Choosing a clinic that offers a special emphasis on women's issues insures that the needs of HIV-infected women will be addressed. Are there processes in place that assure women will get yearly PAP exams, breast exams, and the proper reproductive health counseling? Does the doctor understand the importance of HIV care for the pregnant women? To remain healthy, a woman living with HIV needs a doctor who understands their special needs.

- *Access to Clinical Trials and Studies:* The science of HIV medicine is always advancing. New medicines and treatments have lengthened lives and improved the quality of life for people living with HIV and AIDS. It's important for people living with HIV to have access to the most advanced treatments and medications. Choose a doctor that participates in or has access to clinical trials and studies. As the years pass, having access to clinical trials and cutting edge drugs can mean the difference between chronic illness and long-term health.

- *Choose a Doctor That Encourages Patient Participation:* Insist on a doctor that includes you in all medical decisions and care planning. Studies have shown that patients fare much better if they are participants in their own care. Doctors who empower their patients to make choices in their health care better understand the needs of those living with HIV. Don't consider any doctor or practice that excludes the patient in medical decisions and treatment planning.

The importance of choosing the right doctor for you can't be overstated. The decisions you and your doctor make together will impact your health and quality of life for a very long time. But remember, the doctor you choose does not necessarily need to be your doctor for life. If you find the doctor you choose is just not working out, don't hesitate to look for another. Now that you are infected with HIV, your relationship with your doctor may be the most important relationship you will ever have.

Who Will Manage Your Care?

Chances are you had a family doctor or a primary doctor prior to your HIV diagnosis. That doctor cared for you when you had the flu, a cold, or a fever. Now that you have HIV, you have chosen a doctor to monitor your immune system. What becomes of the doctor that has been caring for you perhaps since you were a child? There are three ways to manage your HIV.

- *Care Managed by Your Family Doctor:* After years of seeing the same family doctor, a trusting doctor-patient relationship develops. After being diagnosed with HIV, the tendency may be to stay with your family doctor and allow him or her to manage your HIV. As discussed earlier, HIV is a very complex disease that requires the expertise only an HIV specialist can provide. For this reason, experts adamantly recommend that HIV not be managed by primary care physicians or family doctors.

- *Care Managed by Your Family Doctor and an HIV Specialist:* A perfectly acceptable way to manage your HIV care is to maintain your family doctor to manage your basic healthcare needs but employ an HIV specialist to manage your HIV and immune system. If you choose this method, make certain that your family doctor and HIV specialist communicate with one another in order to assure continuity of care.

- *Care Managed by an HIV Specialist:* The preferred method of managing your general healthcare and HIV needs is to employ an HIV specialist that can manage both. With one physician managing the whole person, continuity is assured. Having an HIV specialist manage your care does not mean he or she won't refer you to other specialists if needed. If you want to keep your family doctor apprised of your care and condition, make it known to your HIV doctor and he or she can arrange to have regular updates sent to your primary care physician.

Before Your First Visit to the Doctor

Once you have chosen a doctor to manage your HIV, it's time to prepare for that first visit. There are a number of preparations you should make prior to your first visit to the doctor.

- *Get Your Insurance in Order:* To make sure you aren't saddled with a large medical bill, talk to your insurance provider to determine if any referrals are required prior to your first visit. If you don't have insurance coverage, assemble past tax returns, old pay stubs, and a list of your monthly expenses. This information will be needed for you to apply for community resources, Medicaid, and drug assistance programs. Provided the clinic you choose has social worker support, contact them prior to your first visit so they can assist you in getting the insurance coverage you need.

- *Find Your Old Medical Records:* Assemble any old medical records you have, either at home or by asking your family doctor for copies of your past medical record. This will give your new HIV doctor a more complete picture of your medical history prior to your HIV infection.

- *Find a Friend to Come with You:* If possible, arrange to have someone attend your first doctor's appointment with you. Obviously it should be someone you feel comfortable about knowing your diagnosis. That first visit will seem very confusing and overwhelming. It will be extremely helpful to have someone alongside you to help make sense of the large amount of information you are about to receive.
- *Be on Time:* Make certain to arrive to your appointment on time. In fact, arriving a few minutes early is advisable. There will be paperwork that needs to be completed prior to seeing the doctor. Completing the paperwork prior to seeing the doctor allows for more time with the physician. Every minute of your appointment is important. Arriving on time or early makes the best use of the time allotted for your appointment.
- *Bring Plenty of Questions:* Assemble a list of questions for your doctor. Write them down as they occur to you. It's common to forget questions and concerns the minute you walk into the doctor's office. How many times have all of us had a burning question for our doctor, only to forget it the minute we walk into the office? Then, like clockwork, it occurs to us the minute we pull out of the doctor's parking lot. Writing your questions down will insure that they will not be forgotten and will get answered.

Ask the Right Questions

The first thing to keep in mind is that there are no dumb questions. It's essential that you fully understand your HIV treatment plan and how it is formulated by your HIV doctor. So never hesitate to ask questions, and don't leave your doctor's office without the answers you seek.

There are a few questions that you should ask that very first visit to the doctor. It's important to develop a good doctor patient relationship. Just as the doctor asks questions to get to know you better, the answers to your questions will teach you a lot about your doctor and how he or she plans on approaching your HIV care. Asking the right questions not only educates you but also tells your doctor that you have a vested interest in your HIV care and expect to be an active participant from the start. Some important questions to ask your doctor include:

- *Will I be able to play an active role in planning my care and structuring my treatment?*
- *How much time will I have to ask questions at my appointments?*
- *Will I be seen by the same doctor at each visit?*

- *Will I see an attending physician, or will there be resident physicians involved in my doctor visits?*
- *Are walk-in appointments available?*
- *Is there a nurse line I can call if I have an issue that can't wait until my next visit?*
- *Is there a number to call if I have problems after hours and on weekends?*
- *How do you decide what medication regimen is right for me?*
- *Will I have access to clinical trials?*
- *Can I bring a family member, a loved one, or a friend to my visits?*

These are just a few of the most important questions. But, obviously, the questions you ask are specific to your needs. Again, there are no right and wrong questions. In order for you to make sound judgments and decisions, you must have the right answers.

The Ryan White CARE Act

It became evident very early in the epidemic that getting quality medical care soon after diagnosis is the key to living a healthy, productive life with HIV. Unfortunately, the specialty care necessary does not come cheap. While many have the good fortune of medical insurance, a number of HIV-infected people have no medical insurance or the monetary resources to get necessary medical care. In 1990, the United States government passed the Ryan White Comprehensive AIDS Resources Emergency (CARE) Act, providing funds that assure each and every HIV-infected person has access to HIV care.

The Ryan White CARE Act is comprised of several titles that provide funding for specific services. They include:

- *Part A:* This title provides funding to those metropolitan areas (e.g. Detroit, Chicago, San Francisco) hardest hit by HIV and AIDS. The funding provides such services as:
  - Outpatient and ambulatory health services, including substance abuse and mental health treatment;
  - Early intervention that includes outreach, counseling and testing, and referral services designed to identify HIV-positive individuals who are unaware of their HIV status;
  - Outpatient and ambulatory support services including case management; and
  - Inpatient case management services that expedite discharge and prevent unnecessary hospitalization.

- *Part B:* This title provides funding for all fifty states, the District of Columbia, Guam and Puerto Rico. These funds are used for:
    - The AIDS Drug Assistance Program (ADAP);
    - Ambulatory health care;
    - Home-based health care;
    - Insurance coverage;
    - Medications;
    - Support services;
    - Outreach to HIV-positive individuals who know their HIV status;
    - Early intervention services; and
    - The HIV Care Consortia, which assesses needs and contracts for services.
- *Part C:* This title provides funding for primary health care for HIV-infected people. These funds are distributed to such places as free-standing clinics, hospital-based clinics, community health centers, and family planning agencies. The funds provide:
    - Outpatient medical care;
    - Risk-reduction counseling and prevention, antibody testing, medical evaluation, and clinical care;
    - Antiretroviral therapies; protection against opportunistic infections; and ongoing medical, oral health, nutritional, psychosocial, and other care services for HIV-infected clients;
    - Case management to ensure access to services and continuity of care for HIV-infected clients; and
    - Attention to other health problems that occur frequently with HIV infection, including tuberculosis and substance abuse.
- *Part D:* This title provides funding for women, children, and their families. While all titles of the CARE act are required to care for these populations, Title IV funding is specifically for them. This funding provides:
    - Primary and specialty medical care;
    - Psychosocial services;
    - Logistical support and coordination; and
    - Outreach and case management.
- *Special Projects of National Significance (SPNS):* This funding advances knowledge and skills in the delivery of HIV health care. Considered the research portion of the CARE act, it funds a way to:
    - Assess the effectiveness of particular models of care;
    - Support innovative program design; and
    - Promote replication of effective mode.

• *Dental Reimbursement Program*: This title provides funding that supports oral health and dental care for those HIV-infected people without the means or resources to maintain regular dental care.

There are other services and programs not mentioned above that owe their existence to the Ryan White CARE Act, arguably the most important funding available to those people living with HIV and AIDS.

5

Your First Visit to the Doctor

When it's finally time to meet your doctor for the first time, what can you expect? No doubt it will be a very confusing, stressful and frightening time. As you may know, fear is a product of not knowing what to expect. Fear of the unknown can also create stress and anxiety. Knowing what to expect that first visit can help minimize the stress, anxiety and fear. Let's look at the first visit, how to prepare, what to expect, and who you may see.

What You Need to Bring

Getting the most from your doctor's visit requires more than just showing up. You need to prepare for the visit as much as the physician does. There are a few items you should get together and bring with you to that first visit. They include:

- *Your HIV Test Results:* Your doctor will want to review your HIV test results. When you are told of your results by the HIV test counselor, make certain to ask for a copy and bring that copy to your first doctor's visit.
- *Insurance Cards:* If you have insurance coverage, be it private insurance or government assistance, the clerical staff at the doctor's office is going to want to see your insurance cards. Most likely they will make copies of those cards and return them to you by the end of your visit.
- *Insurance Referral:* In this day of Health Management Organizations (HMOs), the insurance referral is very important. HMOs employ a network of physicians from which you can choose to get your care. Every member of the HMO must choose a primary care physician from the network, and it is that physician who must refer you to other specialists, HIV specialists included. Be sure to get a referral prior to your first visit to the HIV specialist, and bring it with you for the clerical staff at the doctor's office. Without a referral some practices will not see you, and at the very least *you* will be billed for your visit instead of your insurance company.

- *Appointment Information:* If you receive an appointment confirmation from your doctor, bring it with you in case there is any confusion surrounding the date or time of your appointment once you arrive at the doctor's office.
- *Old Medical Records:* If you have time prior to your first visit, obtain copies of your past medical records from other physicians who have treated you before your HIV infection. Even medical information not related to your HIV is important to your new doctor. The better he or she knows your past medical history, the better care you will receive now that you have HIV.
- *Questions for Your Doctor:* As was mentioned in a previous chapter, bring a list of any questions you have for your doctor. Because questions can be forgotten easily among all the stress and anxiety of your first visit, write them down as they occur and present that list to your doctor when you arrive. Leave plenty of room on your list for notes and answers to each question.
- *Friend or Loved One for Support:* As mentioned earlier, bringing someone along for emotional support to that first visit will be a great help in digesting the large amount of information you will receive. Obviously, the person you choose should be someone who knows your diagnosis and can offer the assistance and support you need.

TABLE 7

Questions for Your Doctor at Your First Appointment

1. Will I be permitted to play an active role in planning and structuring my care?
2. How much time will I be allotted for questions?
3. Will I be seen by the same doctor each visit?
4. Will I see an attending physician or a resident / student?
5. What days are clinic appointments available?
6. Are "walk-in" appointments available?
7. Is there a nurse-line I can call if my issue can't wait until my next visit?
8. Is there an emergency number I call after hours and on weekends?
9. Will I have access to any experimental treatments or clinical trials?
10. May I bring my partner / spouse / loved one to my visits?

What to Expect Upon Arrival

Most likely, the first people you will encounter at your visit are the clerical staff responsible for registering you for that first visit. Usually, the clerical staff has little medical training but is responsible for getting all the insurance paperwork out of the way before you see the doctor. Normally the staff will ask for your insurance information, any referrals that may be needed, your appointment time, and the name of the physician you are scheduled to see. While the staff is bound by the same confidentiality rules and regulations as the medical personnel, there's no need to provide the check-in staff with details of your diagnosis or medical history. In fact, it's best not to discuss those things in so public an area as the check-in desk. And if you feel the check-in staff are not observing your right to confidentiality, let them know. Once they get you "checked in," your doctor will be notified that you are ready for your appointment. You'll be taken back to an exam room when one becomes available.

What to Expect Once You're in the Exam Room

When an exam room becomes available, you will be escorted to the room by some member of the medical staff. Depending on the type of practice you choose, it may be a medical assistant or a nurse who accompanies you to the room. Once in the room, the nurse or medical assistant will take your blood pressure, heart rate, respiratory rate and temperature.

Many practices will employ registered nurses who make the initial patient contact at each visit. The nurse will usually do a basic assessment to see if there are any complaints, issues, or concerns you would like to pass on to your doctor. Often times the nurse will do a medical history, which includes assessing past and current illnesses, medication history, surgical history, and social history, just to name a few. This is a good time for you the patient to develop a relationship with the nurse. You will find that the nurse will be a very valuable part of your HIV care. Due to the doctor's busy schedule, most often it is the nurse who is available when issues or concerns arise. The nurse is a liaison between you and your doctor. Be upfront and forthright with your concerns and complaints. Many times the doctor relies heavily on what the nurse has learned in the initial assessment. If you leave items out, the doctor may not address them at all during your visit. A good relationship with the nurse will help your relationship with the doctor as well.

When the nurse has completed his or her assessment, the information gained will be forwarded to the physician. Depending on how busy the practice is that day, you may have a short wait in the exam room. Keep an eye out for any educational material available in the room. The time spent waiting can be a valuable learning period if the right educational materials are available. Eventually, it will be your turn to see the doctor.

What to Expect from Your Doctor

The first visit to your doctor will likely be a bit longer than a typical visit once the doctor-patient relationship has been established. At that first visit the doctor is starting with a clean slate, knowing little about you. Much of the visit will be a discussion centering on your past medical history and your current medical condition. This discussion provides your doctor with very important information necessary to provide you the best and most complete medical care. It's important to be honest and forthcoming with facts and information. Some questions the doctor will ask may seem very personal and intrusive. Rest assured that every question has a purpose, so answer each honestly and as completely as possible. Without completely honest answers, pieces of your medical puzzle will be missing, preventing the doctor from providing the medical care you need. If confidentiality is what concerns you, rest assured that physicians and all medical personnel are bound by very strict rules of confidentiality. The information you share with the doctor, nurse or any other person in the medical office remains confidential.

A part of every medical visit is the physical examination. On your first visit, this exam will cover all the body's systems from head to toe. On subsequent visits your doctor will probably limit his physical exam to those systems giving you problems. For instance, if you are having a cough, the doctor will assess and examine your breathing and your lungs. If you are complaining of abdominal pain or nausea, the doctor will examine your stomach. The complete head-to-toe exam performed during the first visit will include:

- *The Head and Neck:* The doctor will examine your head, eyes, and ears. Are you having headaches, visual changes, pain in your ears? The doctor will palpate or feel your neck for any enlarged "glands" or lymph nodes. Enlarged lymph nodes can signal infection. The doctor will also ask if you've had fevers, chills, or night sweats.
- *The Chest:* The doctor will use a stethoscope to listen through your chest and back to assess your lungs. Lung infections such as pneumonia can cause changes in the way your lungs sound when you breathe. The doctor will also use the stethoscope to listen to your heart to see if there are any abnormal heart rhythms or heart sounds that signal illness or disease. Your doctor will also feel under your arms and around your chest for any enlarged lymph nodes. Female patients will get a breast exam to check for any breast lumps that could signal cancer. Finally the doctor will ask if you've had any cough, shortness of breath or chest pain.
- *The Abdomen (stomach):* Using the stethoscope again, the doctor will listen to your abdomen for bowel sounds—the sounds your intestines make when working to digest your food. Again, the doctor will press on your abdomen and your groin, looking for enlarged lymph nodes. He or she will also press on your abdomen to assess if you are having pain or there are any enlarged organs that may indicate illness. Finally, the doctor will ask about your bowel habits, if you've had diarrhea, nausea, or vomiting, if urination is painful, and the color and odor or your urine.
- *Rectal and Genital Areas:* The doctor will do a physical inspection of your genitals and rectal area, looking for any open sores, lumps or lesions that could indicate a sexually transmitted disease. While women will be encour-

aged to have a complete pelvic exam and Pap test by a gynecologist, that exam probably will not be part of your first visit. Men will have a testicular exam to feel for any lumps or masses in the scrotum. The doctor will do a rectal exam by placing a gloved finger in the anus to feel for lumps or masses, and to assess for any blood that may be in the stool. In men, the prostate will be assessed at this time to see if there is any enlargement. Finally, the doctor will ask if you have had any abnormal discharge from the vagina, penis, or anus, as well as any abnormal pain. Female patients will be asked about any past pregnancies, abortions, and miscarriages, as well as questions about the menstrual cycle.

- *Leg, Arms, Hands and Feet:* The upper and lower extremities will be assessed for any swelling or open wounds. The doctor will ask if there is any history of numbness, tingling, or needle-like pain in the hands and feet. Finally the doctor will assess hand and foot strength by having you squeeze his or her hands, and pushing down on his or her hands with your feet.

- *Psychosocial / Mental Status:* The doctor will assess your mental health status by asking a variety of questions. Do you have a history of "passing out"? Do you use alcohol or tobacco? Have you ever abused prescription or recreational drugs? Do you feel depressed or are you having trouble sleeping? Have you ever thought about hurting yourself or hurting others?

- *Sexual and Risk Factor History:* An important part of your first visit's assessment will be a discussion about your risk factors and your sexual history. This allows the doctor to determine how you contracted HIV and to educate you regarding safer sexual practices. Information on the route of transmission is also an important part of tracking the epidemic. The doctor is required to report new infections to the state health department. The information is tabulated by health department staffers and used by prevention specialists in order to target their prevention messages to those populations most at risk.

Who Else Will See You That Day?

Depending on the type of practice you choose, the doctor may not be the only person you will see that first visit. Because HIV affects the whole person, proper HIV care includes many medical and social disciplines. They include:

- *Registered Nurses:* The nurse could be considered the liaison between the doctor and the patient. All practices will have at least one nurse to handle such things as injections, patient teaching, patient telephone calls, and to assist with any office procedures that may be done. In larger practices, the nurse may have his or her own schedule of patients to address issues ranging from medication and adherence teaching to well care visits. Most often the nurse is the medical team member a sick patient will talk to first.

- *Social Workers:* Depending on the practice, social workers play a huge role in the care of the HIV-infected patient. The social worker is primarily responsible for those things not physical in nature, including mental health counseling, the accessing of community resources, and negotiating the medical insurance maze. In addition, social workers play a big role in medication and adherence teaching, HIV prevention, testing and counseling, and safer sex education. Finally, social workers play a very important role in those first few days after diagnosis when the patient is desperately trying to adjust to their new illness.

- *Nutritionists or Dieticians:* Proper diet and nutrition is an important part of staying healthy. If you are fortunate enough to choose a practice that employs a nutritionist, he or she will help you optimize your diet by choosing foods high in the calories and nutrients necessary to fight your illness and remain healthy. The nutritionist can assist with diet and menu planning, exercise programs and medication related-issues surrounding eating and food. Because HIV medicines can cause side effects such as nausea and vomiting, the dietician plays an important role in medication teaching and adherence by instructing the patient in ways to deal with unpleasant medication side effects.

- *Medical Assistants:* Most practices employ medical assistants to handle such tasks as injections, vital signs, and clerical duties. Medical assistants are often responsible for the flow of patients through the clinic, from check-in, to seeing your doctor, to checking out and making the next appointment.

- *Others:* Depending on the type and size of the practice you're part of, there may be several other disciplines involved in your care. Dermatologists to address issues with your skin, dentists to care for your teeth, psychiatrists to address emotional and mental health needs, and pharmacists to assist with medication teaching and adherence education.

Specialty Services

It's inevitable; despite the best medical care, there will be times of poor health. In certain practices, the HIV specialist can also act as the patient's primary care physician, handling such issues as high blood pressure, diabetes, asthma, and the common problems that we all face from time to time. However, there are times when specialists are needed to address illnesses other than HIV. For instance, patients will most likely be referred to a liver specialist (hepatologist) to manage their hepatitis C coinfection. Patients who have heart disease will have a heart specialist (cardiologist) to manage their cardiac problems. Depending on your needs at the time of your first visit, your HIV specialist may refer you to another specialty physician to address concerns not related to HIV.

Now you know what to expect during your first visit to the doctor. Depending on your health status, most doctors will schedule appointments with their patients at least once every three months. Obviously, the number and frequency of visits will change according to your health status. For instance, certain illnesses or changes in medication regimens will require more frequent visits. The purpose of regular visits to your doctor is to keep you healthy. And to do this, there are many blood tests, diagnostic tests, and procedures that help monitor your immune system and overall health. In the next chapter, we will discuss each of these tools in detail.

6

Monitoring Your Health

Obviously, the goal of your HIV care is to stay as healthy as possible for as long as possible. To achieve this goal, your doctor will monitor your health using a variety of tools at his or her disposal. During regular visits, your doctor will physically assess you, using the skills taught during several years of medical training, while using a combination of lab tests, x-rays, and diagnostic procedures to keep tabs on the status of your immune system and your health. This chapter will review the most commonly used of these diagnostic and screening tools.

Blood Tests

At most every visit, your doctor will order an assortment of blood tests to assess the health of your immune system, your endocrine system, your kidneys, and your liver function. Let's look at each test individually.

ELECTROLYTES (LYTES)

Serum electrolytes are substances that circulate in the blood and control the normal function of such things as heart and muscle contraction. Simply put, electrolytes are essential to all bodily functions. While there are several electrolytes in the blood, this test measures the four most important electrolytes, as well as two important indicators of normal kidney function.

- **Sodium (Na):** Sodium is primarily responsible for maintaining osmotic pressure (fluid pressure) within cells and the vascular system. In other words, it maintains a balance between intracellular (fluid inside the cell) and extracellular (fluid outside the cells) fluid levels in the body. Increased serum (blood) sodium is present in states of dehydration resulting from diarrhea or vomiting. Low sodium levels usually are a result of too much fluid within the cells and in the body.
  Normal values: 135 — 145 milliEquivalents/liter (mEq/L)

- **Potassium (K):** Potassium is the major electrolyte involved in heart and muscle function. Even small changes in potassium levels, either too much or too little potassium, can cause abnormal heart rates and rhythms, which in turn negatively impact cardiac (heart) function. Too much potassium in the blood is usually a result of poor kidney function and can adversely affect heart rhythm. Low potassium levels are usually the result of potassium loss resulting from excessive urination or vomiting, and can cause serious changes in heart rhythm.
  Normal values: 3.5–5.0 (mEq/L)
- **Chloride (Cl):** In combination with sodium, chloride maintains fluid levels by regulating osmotic (fluid) pressure in the blood. An elevated chloride level usually results from abnormal kidney function. A chloride level below normal usually results from excessive vomiting or diarrhea.
  Normal values: 100— 106 millimoles/liter (mmol/L)
- **Bicarbonate (HCO3):** Bicarbonate is a substance that helps maintain the proper level of acidity in the blood. If the blood is too acidic or not acidic enough, the body's proper functioning is compromised. The measurement of the blood's acidity is called the pH. Bicarbonate helps make sure the blood pH doesn't get too acidic or not acidic enough. Proper blood pH is essential to life.
  Normal HCO3 values: 35— 45 mmol/L; Normal pH: 7.35— 7.45
- **Blood Urea Nitrogen (BUN):** Urea is a waste product produced in the liver when protein is broken down in the body. Urea is transported via the blood stream to the kidneys where it is excreted. An elevated BUN usually is a result of poor kidney function or inadequate blood circulation to the kidneys. However, BUN is not a good indicator of kidney function because its level can be affected by many things, such as dieting and weight loss.
  Normal values: 8— 25 milligrams/deciliter (mg/dl)
- **Creatinine (Cr):** Creatinine is a waste product formed when muscle tissue uses energy sources found in the body. Creatinine is transported to the kidneys via the blood stream and excreted from the body. Unlike an elevated BUN, elevated creatinine is a very specific indicator of impaired kidney function.
  Normal values: 0.5–1.1 mg/dl

COMPLETE BLOOD COUNT (CBC)

One of the most important blood tests that your doctor will order is the complete blood count (CBC). There are many different types of cells in your blood, and all of them can be grouped into one of three categories: red blood cells, white blood cells, and platelets. This complete blood count helps your doctor determine if your body is trying to fight infection, if your body is able to produce the cells necessary to fight that infection, and if your body is producing an adequate number of the specialized cells that carry oxygen to your organs and tissues.

- **White Blood Cells (WBC):** Also known as leukocytes, white blood cells are produced in the bone marrow and are part of the body's system of fighting infection. An elevated WBC count usually indicates that some type of infection is present and the body is trying to fight it. A count lower than normal suggests that something, a specific medication or a disease process such as HIV, has affected the bone marrow's ability to produce white blood cells. As the WBC count declines, the body's natural defenses against infection grows weaker.
  Normal values: 5000—10000 cells per cubic millimeter of blood
- **Red Blood Cells (RBC):** Also known as erythrocytes, red blood cells are produced by the bone marrow and are responsible for delivering oxygen to tissues and organs throughout the body. As the number of red blood cells declines, so does the body's ability to oxygenate organs and tissues. If the red blood cell count falls too low, organs will fail from lack of oxygen. A low red blood cell count (anemia) can be caused by poor diet and bleeding. In addition, there are certain HIV medications that suppress bone marrow, interfering with red blood cell production, eventually resulting in anemia. Symptoms of anemia include fatigue, pale skin and shortness of breath.
  Normal values: 4.20–5.70 million red cells per microliter of blood
- **Hemoglobin (Hgb):** Hemoglobin is the protein located on the red blood cell that makes it possible for red blood cells to carry oxygen from the lungs to tissues and organs throughout the body. A lower than normal hemoglobin count means the blood's ability to carry oxygen is diminished, impairing all bodily functions. Obviously, without enough oxygen the body begins to fail, causing symptoms such as shortness of breath, chest pain, muscle pain and fatigue. Conditions that cause lower than normal hemoglobin levels include bleeding, diminished red blood cell production by the bone marrow (often a result of certain HIV medications), and poor diet.
  Normal values: Male — 14–17grams of hemoglobin per deciliter of blood (g/dL); Female — 12–15g/dL
- **Hematocrit (Hct):** Whole blood is composed of red blood cells, white blood cells, hemoglobin, platelets, and serum. Hematocrit is a calculated value that represents what percentage of whole blood are red blood cells. A higher than normal hematocrit is most often a result of dehydration that changes the ratio between red blood cells and the fluid portion (serum) of the blood. As the amount of serum decreases, as is the case when a person is dehydrated, the percentage of red blood cells (hematocrit) goes up. Lower than normal hematocrit can be caused by states of fluid overload or

conditions that cause red blood cell production (e.g. decreased bone marrow function, bleeding).

Normal values: Male — 41–50%; Female — 36–44%

- **Platelets (PLT):** Also known as thrombocytes, platelets are produced by the bone marrow and are involved in the blood clotting process. When an opening develops in the vascular system, platelets are dispatched to the area and begin to clump together, forming a plug to seal the breech. Having too few platelets causes prolonged clotting time, which, in extreme cases, can result in severe bleeding. A decreased number of platelets (thrombocytopenia) is usually caused by medications, including certain HIV medications and antibiotics.

Normal values: 140000–390000 platelets per microliter of blood

LIVER FUNCTION TESTS (LFTs)

Liver function tests assess the functioning of the liver by examining the amounts of certain substances in the blood. From these studies, your doctor can identify possible liver disease, medication stress on liver function, or infections of the liver, such as hepatitis. There are several different tests that comprise LFTs.

- **Albumin (ALB):** Albumin is a protein produced by the liver that helps maintain osmotic (fluid) pressure in the vascular space (blood vessels). Albumin helps maintain a pressure balance between the inside and outside of the vessels, assuring that fluid stays in the vascular system instead of leaking out into the tissues, resulting in swelling (edema). Albumin also carries certain minerals in the blood stream. Elevated albumin levels usually indicate dehydration, while lower than normal albumin levels can indicate liver dysfunction or insufficient protein intake.

Normal values: 4–6 grams per deciliter of blood (g/dl)

- **Alkaline Phosphatase (ALK PHOS):** Alkaline phosphatase is an enzyme found in many organs of the body, including the liver. This enzyme is released into the bloodstream when liver tissue damage has occurred. While lower than normal alkaline phosphatase levels are not significant, elevated levels indicate liver dysfunction and liver tissue damage.

Normal values: 30–120 units per liter of liter (U/L)

- **Alanine Aminotransferase (ALT or SGPT):** This protein is found primarily in the liver. It is released into the blood when there has been some sort of liver tissue damage. While lower than normal levels are really insignificant, elevated levels result when there has been liver tissue damage as a result of infection, medications, chemicals, obstruction, cirrhosis or injury to the liver.

Normal values: Less than 35 U/L

- **Aspartate Aminotransferase (AST or SGOT):** This protein is found primarily in the liver. It is released into the blood when there has been some sort of liver tissue damage. Like ALT, lower than normal levels are not significant, but elevated levels result when there has been liver tissue damage caused by infection, medicines, obstructions, cirrhosis, chemicals, or injury to the liver.
  Normal values: less than 35 U/L
- **Total Bilirubin (TBILI):** Bilirubin is a normal component of red blood cells. When these cells break down, free bilirubin is released into the blood. Bilirubin is then carried to the liver, where it is broken down and excreted. When the liver is not functioning properly, bilirubin builds up in the body, causing jaundice (yellowing of the skin and eyes, and darkening of the urine). Elevated bilirubin is caused by a dysfunction of the system that breaks down bilirubin, which includes the liver. Such an elevation can be caused by an obstruction, liver disease or liver failure. HIV medicines can cause a harmless elevation of total bilirubin by interfering with the system that removes bilirubin from the blood.
  Normal values: less than 1.0 milligrams/deciliter of blood (mg/dl)
- **Unconjugated Bilirubin (BU):** Also known as indirect bilirubin, unconjugated bilirubin is a type of bilirubin that is not water soluble. Bilirubin needs to be water soluble in order to be excreted through the urine. Unconjugated bilirubin is carried to the liver by albumin and is then transformed to a water soluble form with the help of special enzymes. Elevated BU can occur with many blood disorders, liver disease, or resolution of large blood clots. An elevated BU can also be caused by one specific protease inhibitor know as Reyataz (atazanavir). More on HIV medications will come in a later chapter.
  Normal values: less than 1.0 mg/dl
- **Conjugated Bilirubin (BC):** Conjugated bilirubin is the water soluble form of bilirubin. Elevated conjugated bilirubin is indicative of impaired liver function, and can signal impending liver failure.
  Normal values: less than 1.0 mg/dl

CHOLESTEROL AND TRIGLYCERIDE PROFILE

Cholesterol and triglycerides are substances produced naturally in the body. However, much of the foods we eat are sources of cholesterol and triglycerides. Because of their impact on the health of the heart, pancreas, and liver, it is important to monitor cholesterol and triglycerides in the blood.

- **Cholesterol:** There are two sources of cholesterol — the cholesterol your body produces naturally and the cholesterol present in animal products that you eat (fish, meats, eggs, and poultry). In addition, certain foods that don't contain cholesterol do contain fatty acids that the body uses to produce more cholesterol. Certain disease processes, as well as certain medications, can cause cholesterol levels to rise. Because elevated cholesterol has been associated with heart disease, it is important to monitor cholesterol levels on a regular basis, especially in people living with diseases that have been associated with increased risk of heart disease, such as HIV. While there are other causes, usually elevated cholesterol is a result of a diet high in cholesterol-containing foods.

Normal values:
- *Desirable — less than 200 mg/dl*
- *Borderline High Risk — 201 to 239 mg/dl*
- *High Risk — greater than 240 mg/dl*

• **Triglycerides:** Fats that are taken into the body as part of the diet are used as an energy source. However, if more fat is taken in than is needed by the body for energy, the excessive fat is stored in the body as triglycerides. A triglyceride blood test can measure how much of the fatty substance is in circulation. Any excess triglycerides not immediately used for energy are stored in the body as adipose (fat) tissue. Meals high in fatty foods, and consuming alcohol, raise the triglyceride level in the blood. In addition, some HIV medications can dramatically elevate triglyceride levels, so much so that lipid-lowering medication is required to bring triglyceride levels down. While there are many causes of elevated triglycerides, most often, elevated triglycerides are related to a diet of fatty foods.

Normal values: 90–150 mg/dl

• **High-density lipoprotein cholesterol (HDL):** This type of cholesterol is known as the "good cholesterol." Like cholesterol, the level of HDL is primarily related to diet. Higher levels of HDL have been shown to decrease the risk of heart disease. Some studies have shown that HDL slows the build-up of cholesterol in blood vessels. It's this build-up that narrows and eventually occludes the vessels that supply the heart muscle with blood. Without blood, the heart muscle is damaged, diminishing the heart's ability to pump blood throughout the body. In other words, when a vessel becomes occluded, the person suffers a heart attack. Its ability to slow the build-up of cholesterol is why HDL is known as the good cholesterol.

Normal values: Male — 44 mg/dl; Female — 55 mg/dl

• **Low-density lipoprotein cholesterol (LDL):** This type of cholesterol is known as the "bad cholesterol" because excessive amounts will slowly build up along the inner walls of blood vessels. In combination with other substances present, LDL forms plaque, the hard substance that build up on the vessel walls and eventually causes blockages that stop blood flow to the heart muscle. Like most cholesterol, LDL level is primarily dependant on diet.

Normal values:
- *Desirable — less than 130 mg/dl*
- *Borderline High Risk — 131–160 mg/dl*
- *High Risk — greater than 160 mg/dl*

Monitoring Your Immune System ... Monitoring Your HIV

As mentioned in an earlier chapter, the key to staying healthy is frequent monitoring of your immune system. The presence of opportunistic infections, illnesses, or cancers does signal a weakening immune system, but wouldn't it be better to know the immune system is weak before getting sick? Recognizing a weakened immune system or active HIV replication before a person gets sick is an important step in keeping a person healthy for a longer period of time. There are blood tests that monitor your immune system strength and the activity of your HIV.

CD4 Cells (T-cells)

T-cells (or T-lymphocytes) are specialized types of white blood cells that play an important role in the immune system. There are two main types of T-cells, one of which has molecules on their surface called CD4. These "helper" cells orchestrate the body's defensive response to microorganisms such as viruses. The other type of T-cell has molecules called CD8 on their surface that destroy infected cells by producing antiviral substances. Unfortunately, HIV is able to attach itself to the CD4 molecule, allowing the virus to enter and infect T-cells, damaging them in the process. The CD4 count is a reflection of how many functional CD4 T-cells are circulating in the blood. Your doctor can assess the health of your immune system and its ability to fight off infection by monitoring the number of healthy CD4 cells. Your doctor will monitor your CD4 count often — at least every three months, and more often if you are sick or have recently started a new drug regimen.

Normal values:
- In the absence of HIV: 500 to 1500 CD4 cells per cubic millimeter of blood
- In the HIV-infected person:
  - Minimum Goal — greater than 200
  - Desired — greater than 500
  - Consider Medications — less than 350

HIV Viral Load

The HIV viral load blood test measures the number of active HIV copies in a milliliter of blood. Scientific evidence has proven that keeping the HIV viral load as low as possible for as long as possible decreases the complications of HIV disease. It makes sense. HIV attacks CD4 cells, damaging them and weakening the immune system in the process. As the immune system weakens, the body becomes more at risk for infections and sickness. By keeping the HIV viral load low, fewer CD4 cells are damaged and the immune system stays strong and able to fight infection and illness. Your doctor will monitor your HIV viral load on a regular basis—at least every three months, and more often if you are sick or have recently begun a new medication regimen. By measuring the number of active HIV copies in circulation, your doctor can assess several things:

- *The status of your HIV disease:* Is your HIV under control? Is your current HIV regimen working? Are you at risk for disease progression and opportunistic infections?
- *The predicted course of your disease:* Will your disease progress rapidly or slowly? Will you be at risk for opportunistic infections in the future? Will your disease respond to your current or future regimens?
- *What medication regimen will work for you:* Is this regimen working? If not, which regimens will work? Do you need to be on medications at all?

What Does the Viral Load Result Mean?

As mentioned above, the HIV viral load measures the number of HIV copies in a milliliter of blood. The greater the number, the more copies of active virus are present. As the number of active virus increases, so does the damage done to CD4 cells in the immune system.

The HIV viral load can be measured with many different types of tests. It is important to use the same type of test each time the viral load is measured. Most of the time, your doctor will use one of two HIV viral load tests.

- **Quantitative HIV Viral Load:** This viral load test is the least sensitive of the two, measuring viral load from greater than 400 HIV copies per milliliter of blood to less than 750,000 HIV copies per milliliter of blood. People with values less than 400 are said to have an *undetectable* viral load. Keep in mind that undetectable means that the number of HIV copies is fewer than the test's ability to measure. It does not mean that there are no copies of HIV present. Unfortunately, that can't be achieved with the currently available treatments. This test is used for people suspected to have viral load counts greater than one thousand.
- **Ultrasensitive HIV Viral Load:** This test is the more sensitive of the two viral load tests, measuring a viral load from greater than 48 to less than 75,000. Actually, newer viral load tests can measure viral loads as high as 10,000,000. People with viral load values less than 48 are said to have an undetectable viral load. This test is primarily for people suspected of having an HIV viral load less than 1000.

Interpreting Results

As mentioned above, there is no way to completely eradicate HIV from the body. However, the fewer HIV copies the better. Results will be reported as follows:

- **Undetectable:** Less than 48 (<48), using the ultrasensitive HIV viral load test; or less than 400 (<400), using the quantitative HIV viral load test. Undetectable means that the number of circulating HIV copies is less than the test's ability to measure.

- **Detectable:** This value is reported as the number of HIV copies per milliliter of blood. The values range from greater than 48 to less than 10 million copies (51–10,000,000), using the ultrasensitive test; and greater than 400 to less than 750,000 copies (401–750,000), using the quantitative HIV viral load test. Results greater than 75,000 (>75,000) or 750,000 (>750,000) means there are so many HIV copies present they exceed the test's ability to measure the exact number of HIV copies present.

Your doctor uses the HIV viral load results to determine if you need to begin medicines or to assess how well the current drug regimen is working. While the guidelines change frequently, at the time of this printing, a person with an HIV viral load greater than 100,000 may be a candidate for HIV medications. All the factors used to determine if a person needs HIV therapy will be discussed in more detail in a later chapter.

HIV GENOTYPE TEST

One of the characteristics that makes HIV such a formidable disease is its ability to change and mutate in response to medications. After prolonged exposure to an HIV treatment regimen, the virus has the ability to change its genetic structure (mutate) in a way that makes it resistant to the medication regimen being taken. Eventually, the regimen must be changed in order to effectively control HIV replication. But how does your doctor know which regimen will be effective after the virus has mutated? The HIV genotype test can assist the doctor in choosing a new medication regimen that will be effective.

With the assistance of the HIV genotype test, HIV mutations are identified and medication regimens are chosen accordingly. The presence of certain types of mutations mean certain medications will no longer be effective in preventing HIV replication. Certain mutations are associated with certain medications. For instance, there is a certain mutation that is very specific to the HIV medication Epivir, meaning that if that mutation is present, Epivir will no longer be effective. To go one step further, certain mutations can mean resistance to entire classes of drugs, not just individual medications. By examining your HIV with the genotype test, your doctor knows which medicines will and will not work, enabling him or her to put together a medication regimen that's right for you.

HIV PHENOTYPE TESTING

As mentioned earlier, HIV can change or mutate, making the choice of an HIV medication regimen at times very difficult. A less frequently used blood test that can help your doctor choose an effective therapy is an HIV phenotype. Unlike the genotype test, which identifies resistance by looking at viral mutations, phenotype testing actually exposes the virus to individual drugs, identifying which have the greatest effect and control viral replication best. That information makes it possible for the doctor to choose a drug regimen containing medications proven by the phenotype test to be effective against the type of virus present.

Other Important Blood Tests

While not as routine as the blood tests discussed earlier in this chapter, the following blood tests are very important in assessing the health status and medical needs of people living with HIV.

HEPATITIS SEROLOGIES

Like any other part of the body, the liver can acquire infections or be damaged when exposed to such things as chemicals, medications, bacteria, viruses, parasites, or alcohol. What results is an inflammation of the liver known as hepatitis. As we know from an earlier discussion, there are liver function studies that can identify inflammation and damage that has occurred to the liver. There are also blood tests that can identify specific causes of hepatitis. For instance, there are several viral types of hepatitis, each needing different approaches to treatment and cure. For this reason it is important to identify which virus type is causing the hepatitis. While there are several different types of viral hepatitis, the three most common are hepatitis A, hepatitis B, and hepatitis C.

- **Hepatitis A (HAV):** This type of viral infection is primarily spread from person to person by way of contaminated food or water. Two blood tests are used to identify hepatitis A, both looking for hepatitis A antibodies. A positive result of either test means that the person has been exposed to hepatitis A. The two tests are:
    - IgM antibody to HAV (IgM anti–HAV)
    - Total antibody to HAV (total anti–HAV)
- **Hepatitis B (HBV):** This viral infection is spread from person to person by exposure to contaminated blood by way of needle sticks, open wounds,

or lacerations. There are five markers tested for to identify hepatitis b infection, some more sensitive than others. These markers seek to identify hepatitis b proteins or antibodies to hepatitis b that the body has produced after exposure to the virus. Interpretation of these results can be tricky, dependant upon medical history and the clinical setting.

- Hepatitis B surface antigen (HBsAg)
- Hepatitis B core antigen (HBeAg)
- Hepatitis B core antibody (anti–HBe)
- Hepatitis B surface antibody (anti–HBs)—*note: will be positive after hepatitis B vaccination*
- Hepatitis B viral load (Hepatitis B DNA PCR): This test measures the amount of active hepatitis B virus present in a blood sample. This test is the most sensitive available for the diagnosis of hepatitis B infection.

• **Hepatitis C (HCV):** This viral infection is transmitted primarily through exposure to contaminated blood or blood products by way of needle sticks and sharing needles to inject drugs. HCV infection is rapidly becoming a disease of epidemic proportions. A positive HCV test result confirms the presence of antibodies to hepatitis C (anti–HCV) and allows for diagnosis.

- Hepatitis C viral load (HCV PCR): The most sensitive measure of hepatitis C, this test measures the amount of active virus present in a sample of blood.

IDENTIFYING PAST AND PRESENT INFECTIONS

Blood tests can be used to identify active infections or those infections that have been resolved but have left antibodies behind. When treating HIV, obviously it is important to identify current infections. However, being aware of past infections is also important for maintaining optimal health. Here are some of the most common tests used to identify past and present infections.

• **Cytomegalovirus (CMV):** A majority of adults have been exposed to CMV, a member of the herpes family, at some point in their lifetime. In the person with a normal functioning immune system, CMV most often exhibits few if any symptoms. However, in a person living with HIV, the damaged immune system is not able to fight CMV, which can result in serious illness. This blood test identifies the presence of CMV antibody, which confers past exposure and/or infection with CMV.

• **Toxoplasmosis (Toxo; TPM):** Caused by the parasite *Toxoplasma gondii*, this serious infection is usually spread to humans by way of undercooked meat and poorly prepared or contaminated food. Blood tests can identify antibodies that result from an active infection, while other tests can be done to identify past toxoplasma infections.

- **Herpes Simplex (HSV):** There are actually two types of HSV — HSV-1, which is responsible for oral and facial herpes, and HSV-2, which is responsible for genital herpes. Differentiation between the two is very difficult but possible using antibody blood tests. HSV is transmitted by sexual contact and can cause serious illness, especially in people living with HIV. Viral cultures of existing lesions can also identify HSV.

BLOOD CULTURES

Anyone with a weakened immune system, including those living with HIV, are at risk for systemic infections—those infections that spread from a localized area to the entire body. Systemic infections (for instance, those infections in the blood stream) can cause serious illness. To identify the organisms that cause these types of infections, blood is drawn and placed in special growth media. After several days, the media is examined for any organisms that have grown. The presence of organisms in the blood sample confirms the type of systemic infection. Once organisms are identified, the appropriate treatment can be initiated. The testing process used to grow and identify these infectious organisms is called a *blood culture.*

TUBERCULOSIS (TB) SCREENING—PPD

While not a blood test, TB screening relies on the presence of antibodies to identify past and current infection with tuberculosis. Just as blood tests identify the presence of antibodies from past infections, the TB test relies on the antibody response to identify past TB exposure and infection. It's an important tool in maintaining the health of the HIV-infected individual.

The test consists of a very small amount of *mycobacterium tuberculosis* (TB), Purified Protein Derivative (PPD), being injected just under the skin. If the person has been exposed to TB in their lifetime, the antibodies would be present in the body. The PPD injected under the skin is detected by existing TB antibodies, causing a localized itching, redness, and swelling that signals an antibody response to the PPD, confirming past exposure to TB. Keep in mind that in order for an antibody response to occur, the immune system must be in working order, a requirement that makes TB tests unreliable at times with the weakened immune system of the person living with HIV. A more detailed explanation of TB will appear in a later chapter.

Radiology Studies

In addition to the variety of blood tests that are done, there are many radiological studies ("x-rays") used to monitor and maintain your health. Most often these x-rays are ordered in response to symptoms of illness. They are, however, also done to establish a baseline for comparison purposes if future symptoms arise. Some of the most common radiology tests include:

- *Chest X-ray:* As the name implies, a chest x-ray is a picture of the chest and the lungs using electromagnetic radiation to cast an image on a photographic plate. This technology makes it possible to examine the lungs and other internal features without opening the body. The chest x-ray is used primarily to detect fluid collections that result from a variety of lung infections, such as bacterial pneumonia or pneumocystis pneumonia (PCP). Other uses of the chest x-ray included identifying rib fractures, heart size, degree of lung expansion, and the presence of tuberculosis (TB).

- *Abdominal X-ray:* As the name suggests, this is an x-ray of the abdominal cavity. While x-rays don't provide the best picture of the stomach and intestinal tract, they do identify air and fluid collections in the abdominal cavity. The presence of air or fluid is important to identify because both conditions suggest infection, abscess or perforation of the bowel. Some abdominal x-rays require patients to drink special liquids prior to taking the x-rays. These liquids don't allow x-rays to pass through them (*radio opaque*), thereby outlining the intestines and stomach, providing a more accurate exam. Most often, if an abnormality is found with an abdominal x-ray, more accurate and sensitive studies are done to confirm the results.

- *Computed Axial Tomography Scan (CT scan):* To better understand what a CT scan is, think of a fruitcake. Looking at the outside it would be impossible to imagine how complex the inside is—nuts, different kinds of fruit, the cake itself. If you took a knife and cut a slice, you could see the outside as well as the complexity of the inside of the cake. In a sense, that's exactly what a CT scan does, but instead of using a knife, the slices are done with x-rays. A CT scan creates "x-ray slices" of the body, allowing doctors to see what is going on inside the body without actually cutting the body as you would a fruitcake. The resulting pictures are much more accurate, and contain much greater detail, than conventional x-rays. The increased resolution and accuracy of a CT scan allows for earlier and more accurate diagnosis. CT scans are used on almost every part of the body, but most often on the brain, the sinuses, the chest and the abdomen.

- *Magnetic Resonance Imaging (MRI):* Technically, an MRI is not a type of x-ray at all. Instead, radio waves and strong magnetic fields are used to take very detailed images of the body's internal structure. The MRI is used primarily to take high resolution images of the brain, spinal cord, abdomen and chest in order to identify infection, inflammation, fluid collections, or masses. Just as CT scans confirm the findings of general x-rays, MRIs often confirm those findings of CT scans. MRIs are able to produce much more detailed still images and moving pictures when compared to those produced by CT scans.

- *Positron Emission Tomography (PET scan):* PET scans use radioactive substances to identify abnormal tissue in the body — specifically, cancerous cells. A normal body substance, most often glucose, is "tagged" with a radioactive substance. This glucose is then injected into a vein and allowed to circulate throughout the body. After about forty five minutes, the patient is placed in a scanner that locates areas in the body where the radioactive-tagged glucose has accumulated. Cancerous cells "take up" more of the radioactive glucose than normal tissue, causing cancerous tissue to appear brighter when compared to normal tissue. This characteristic of cancerous cells makes it possible to identify cancer by the amount of tagged glucose that has accumulated. While the PET scan is not used as often as a CT scan or an MRI, it is a very useful tool in identifying cancers such as lymphoma in HIV-infected people.

Now that we know what tools your doctor will use to monitor your health and the health of your immune system, let's look at the medications used to treat your HIV. After all, it is the HIV medications that prevent you from getting serious opportunistic infections that can rob you of your health and eventually your life.

7

Know Your HIV Medications

During the first five years of the HIV/AIDS epidemic, people diagnosed with the disease died within a few months. Simply put, AIDS was a death sentence. In 1987 the FDA approved the first medication to treat HIV, providing new hope for everyone touched by this disease. Five years later the strongest of all HIV medications, the protease inhibitors, were developed, and death rates started to decline for the first time since the epidemic began.

It's no secret that the medications have made HIV a disease people live with, not die from. But for the medications to do their job, people living with HIV must be educated about how they work, how they must be taken, and the importance of adhering to prescribed regimens. This chapter discusses HIV medicines, delineates why adherence is important, provides ideas that will help you better adhere to your regimen, and discusses side effects you may experience. But first, to understand HIV medicines, we must understand the HIV life cycle. Attacking HIV at many points in its life cycle is the key to the effectiveness of HIV medications. Let's review the HIV life cycle.

The HIV Life Cycle

Chapter 3 introduced the HIV life cycle in detail. Now, to better understand how each class of HIV medication works, let's review what we learned in chapter 3 with the addition of each class of HIV medication and how it interrupts the life cycle.

INTRODUCTION OF HIV INTO THE BODY

Obviously, before the HIV life cycle can begin, HIV must enter the body. As we learned earlier, exposure to infected bodily fluids during sexual contact or by sharing needles is the primary means by which HIV enters the body. While less common, HIV can also enter the body during pregnancy, child birth or by ingesting HIV-infected breast milk.

Viral Attachment

Once in the body, HIV needs to attach to CD4 cells in order to replicate. While no medications are currently available to prevent this attachment, there are trials and research being conducted on proteins that inhibit viral attachment. This research could lead to medications that would inhibit viral attachment. It's believed that interrupting viral attachment will stop HIV replication in its tracks, and, in turn, will preserve CD4 cells and the immune system.

Viral Fusion

Once attached to the cell, HIV injects its own proteins into the cellular fluids (cytoplasm) of the human CD4 cell. This causes a *fusion* or joining of the human host cell membrane to the outer envelope of the HIV particle. Currently there is one class of drug that interrupts viral fusion — the *Fusion Inhibitor*. Fusion inhibitors prevent viral fusion, thereby interrupting the HIV life cycle and impeding HIV replication.

The Uncoating

In order for HIV to use its genetic material (RNA) for reproduction, the protective coating surrounding the RNA strand must be dissolved. Not much is known about this step, but one thing is certain — without this step, conversion of HIV RNA to DNA can't take place, and replication is halted. Currently, research is being done in hopes of finding a way to inhibit HIV from shedding this protective coating. If a way can be found, it could lead to an entirely new class of HIV medication.

Reverse Transcription

Once in the cell, the single-stranded HIV RNA must be converted to double-stranded DNA. This takes place with the help of the enzyme *reverse transcriptase*. Reverse transcriptase uses proteins from the CD4 cell to help change the HIV RNA to HIV DNA. Reverse transcriptase allows genetic information to flow in the opposite direction (RNA to DNA), as opposed to the normal direction (DNA to RNA). The resulting DNA contains the viral genetic information needed for HIV replication to continue to the next step.

Two classes of HIV medications interrupt the reverse transcription stage by inhibiting reverse transcriptase.

- *Nucleoside Reverse Transcriptase Inhibitors (NRTIs)* are medications that contain faulty imitations of nucleotides found in CD4 cells. Instead of incorporating a cellular nucleotide into the growing chain of DNA, the imitation building block provided by the NRTI is inserted, preventing the double strand of DNA from becoming fully formed and formed correctly.

- *Non-nucleoside Reverse Transcriptase Inhibitors (NNRTIs)* are medications that block reverse transcription by attaching to the reverse transcriptase enzyme in a way that prevents it from functioning normally.

INTEGRATION

To use the cell during replication, HIV must *integrate* or insert its newly formed DNA into the CD4 cell's nucleus. The nucleus is the brain of the cell, containing all of the RNA and DNA of that cell. Integration of viral DNA into the nucleus is accomplished with the help of a special protein called an enzyme; in this case, the enzyme is called *retroviral integrase.* Enzymes start and fuel chemical reactions. In the case of the HIV life cycle, retroviral integrase fuels the chemical reaction that inserts the viral DNA into the CD4 cell.

VIRAL LATENCY

Webster's Dictionary defines latency as an incubation period or a period of waiting. HIV must wait for additional proteins to be manufactured before replication can be completed. This period of waiting is known as viral latency.

FINAL ASSEMBLY

Once the viral proteins are manufactured, they must be cut into pieces and assembled into new HIV particles. This *cleavage* or cutting is accomplished with the help of another protein enzyme called *protease.* The protease enzyme cuts the proteins into smaller pieces, allowing those pieces to reassemble into new HIV particles.

There is a class of HIV medication that interrupts this stage of the HIV life cycle by inhibiting the enzyme protease. *Protease Inhibitors* bind to the protease enzyme and prevent it from separating or cleaving into smaller pieces. Without cleavage, HIV can't be assembled. The protease inhibitors that interfere with viral cleavage are considered the most potent of all the HIV medications.

BUDDING

Budding is the final step in the HIV life cycle. The newly formed HIV particle, complete with viral genetic material and a new outer coat made from the cell membrane of the human host CD4 cell, "pinches off" of the host cell and enters the body's circulation. After a period of *maturation,* a "growing up" so to speak, the newly formed HIV is ready to attach to another CD4 cell and start the process all over again. There are no drugs available that interrupt this final stage, but current studies are showing that a new class of drug, the *Maturation Inhibitor,* has great promise in the fight against HIV.

HIV Medication Drug Classes

Now that we have taken a brief look at how each drug class fits into the HIV life cycle, let's take a closer, more detailed look at each class and the drugs that comprise them.

ENTRY INHIBITORS

Entry inhibitors interfere with the fusion of HIV to the human CD4 cell it needs to replicate. There are areas on the outer surface of HIV (CCR5, CXCR4) that makes it possible for HIV to fuse to the CD4 cell. As part of the HIV life cycle, chemical structural changes occur allowing HIV to attach to the CD4. Drugs in this class interrupt the attachment of HIV to the CD4 cell.

- Fuzeon (enfuvirtide) — Roche Laboratories Inc. and Trimeris Inc.
- Selzentry (maraviroc) — Pfizer

PROTEASE INHIBITORS

During the final assembly stage of the HIV life cycle, the viral proteins must be "cut up" or cleaved into the smaller pieces that are later assembled into the new HIV particle. The enzyme protease is an essential part of this step of cleavage and reassembling. Protease inhibitors block the enzyme protease, interfering with cleavage and assembly, thereby interrupting the HIV life cycle. There are currently nine protease inhibitors available:

- Aptivus (tipranavir) — Boehringer Ingelheim
- Crixivan (indinavir) — Merck
- Fortovase (saquinavir) — Roche Laboratories (*at the time of this printing, Fortovase was scheduled to be discontinued and replaced by Invirase*)
- Invirase (saquinavir) — Roche Laboratories
- Kaletra (lopinavir + ritonavir) — Abbott Laboratories
- Lexiva (fosamprenavir) — GlaxoSmithKline
- Norvir (ritonavir) — Abbott Laboratories
- Prezista (darunavir) — Tibotec
- Reyataz (atazanavir) — Bristol-Meyers Squibb
- Viracept (nelfinavir) — Pfizer

Note that the protease inhibitor Fortovase (saquinavir soft gel capsule) will be discontinued early in 2006 and replaced with the more popular formulation of Invirase (saquinavir hard gel cap).

NUCLEOSIDE REVERSE TRANSCRIPTASE INHIBITORS

A very important stage in the HIV life cycle involves the transfer of HIV genetic material into the CD4 cell. This essential step can't occur without the enzyme *reverse transcriptase*. The *Nucleoside Reverse Transcriptase Inhibitors* (*NRTIs*) are medications that contain faulty imitations of nucleotides (proteins) found in CD4 cells. During genetic transfer, the imitation building block provided by the NRTI is inserted into the growing DNA chain. These faulty proteins prevent the double strand of DNA from forming correctly. The resulting DNA strand is flawed, preventing effective HIV replication. Currently there are thirteen NRTIs available. They include:

- Viread (tenofovir) — Gilead
- Combivir (lamivudine + zidovudine) — GlaxoSmithKline
- Epivir (lamivudine) — GlaxoSmithKline
- Zerit (stavudine) — Bristol-Myers Squibb
- Hivid (zalcitabine) — Roche Laboratories
- Videx EC (didanosine) — Bristol-Meyers Squibb
- Retrovir (AZT, zidovudine) — GlaxoSmithKline
- Ziagen (abacavir) — GlaxoSmithKline
- Trizivir (lamivudine + zidovudine + abacavir) — GlaxoSmithKline
- Emtriva (emtricitabine) — Gilead
- Epzicom (lamivudine + abacavir) — GlaxoSmithKline
- Truvada (tenofovir + emtricitabine) — Gilead

NON-NUCLEOSIDE REVERSE TRANSCRIPTASE INHIBITORS (NNRTI)

Very similar to the NRTIs are the *Non-nucleoside Reverse Transcriptase Inhibitors*. Like NRTIs, the NNRTIs interrupt the HIV life cycle by blocking the enzyme reverse transcriptase. However, the mechanism by which NNRTIs block reverse transcriptase differs from NRTIs. Non-nucleoside reverse transcriptase inhibitors (NNRTIs) work by attaching to the reverse transcriptase enzyme, blocking its normal function. Without properly functioning reverse transcriptase, HIV replication is impeded. Currently there are three NNRTIs available:

- Sustiva (efavirenz) — Bristol-Myers Squibb
- Viramune (neviripine) — Boehringer Ingelheim
- Rescriptor (delavirdine) — Pfizer

INTEGRASE INHIBITORS

Integrase is an enzyme that does what the name implies; it integrates HIV genetic material into the DNA of human CD4 cells, making it possible for the infected cell to make new copies of HIV. By interfering with integrase during the HIV life cycle, the integrase inhibitors prevent HIV genetic material from integrating into the CD4 cell, thus stopping viral replication.

- Isentress (raltegravir)—Merck

Numerous studies have provided data and statistics that prove beyond a shadow of a doubt that HIV medications are effective. However, studies also show they are not always easy to take. The key to an affective treatment regimen is the ability to take the medications on time each and every day while missing very few, if any, doses. By knowing as much about your medications as possible, taking them becomes much easier. The following tables provide medication information that will help you better understand the medications you are taking.

More about Medications — Doses / Frequency / Side Effects

FUSION INHIBITORS / CCR5 INHIBITORS / INTEGRASE INHIBITORS

Medication	Forms	Dose	How to take	Side Effects	Interactions
Fuzeon (enfuvirtide)	Reconstituted powder	90mg twice daily	Subcutaneous injection	Injection site reactions	
Selzentry (Maraviroc)	150mg and 300mg tablets	300mg twice daily	Can be taken with or without food about 12 hours apart	Cough, fever, upper respiratory infections, rash, sore muscles, abdominal pain, dizziness, heart problems, elevated liver enzymes	No known drug interactions
Isentress (raltegravir)	400mg tablets	400mg twice daily	Can be taken with or without food about 12 hours apart	The most common are headache and diarrhea	

PROTEASE INHIBITORS

Medication	Forms	Dose	How to take	Side Effects	Interactions
Aptivus (tipranavir)	250mg soft gel capsules	2 capsules twice each day	Must be taken with Norvir 200mg twice each day	Nausea, vomiting, diarrhea, rash, jaundice	Should not be taken with Viagra, St. John's Wort
Crixivan (indinavir)	400mg capsules	2 capsules three times each day	Must drink at least 2 liters of water each day; take on empty stomach	Back pain, blood in urine (both symptoms of kidney stones)	Should not be taken with Viagra, St. John's Wort
Fortovase / Invirase (saquinavir)	200mg soft and hard gel capsules; 500mg tablet	(6) 200mg soft capsules three times daily; (5) 200mg hard gel capsules twice daily; (2) 500mg tablets twice daily	500mg tablets must be taken with 100mg Norvir twice each day; take on full stomach	Nausea, vomiting, diarrhea, burning in feet or hands	Should not be taken with Viagra, St. John's Wort, Rifampin or Rifabutin *Fortovase was discontinued in early 2006
Kaletra (lopinavir + ritonavir)	Soft gel capsules with 133mg lopinavir and 33mg ritonavir; Tablets containing 200mg lopinavir and 50mg ritonavir	(3) capsules twice daily; (4) capsules twice daily if taken with Sustiva or Viramune; (2) tablets twice daily; *Soft gel capsules can be taken as 6 capsules once daily	Soft gel capsules should be taken with food; Tablets can be taken with or without food	Fatigue, headache, nausea, vomiting, diarrhea, elevated cholesterol & triglycerides	Should not be taken with Viagra, St. John's Wort. Not to be taken with Norvir capsules

Medication	Forms	Dose	How to take	Side Effects	Interactions
Lexiva (fosamprenavir)	700mg tablets	(1) tablet with Norvir twice daily; (2) tablets twice daily; (2) tablets and 200mg Norvir twice daily	Take with or without food	Malaise, headache, nausea, diarrhea, vomiting, loss of appetite, elevated triglycerides & cholesterol	Should not be taken with Viagra, St. John's Wort
Norvir (ritonavir)	100mg soft gel capsules	Used in various doses as a boosting agent for other PIs	Take with food, preferably high fat meals	Abdominal pain, nausea, vomiting	Should not be taken with Viagra, St. John's Wort; no longer a lone agent
Prezista (darunavir)	300mg and 600mg tablets	(2) 300mg tablets or 600mg tablets with 100mg Norvir twice daily	Take with food and store at room temperature	Nausea, diarrhea, common cold symptoms, rash	

If you take any of these drugs notify your doctor:
- erectile dysfunction drugs such as Viagra
- drugs to treat TB
- drugs to control abnormal heart rhythms
- migraine headache medications
- antihistamines
- antifungal meds
- birth control pills
- methadone
- buprenorphine
- St. John's Wort

Medication	Forms	Dose	How to take	Side Effects	Interactions
Reyataz (atazanavir)	150mg and 200mg capsules	(2) 200mg capsules once each day; (2) 150mg capsules when boosted with 100mg Norvir	Take with food; When using boosted dose, take at the same time as Norvir	Nausea, vomiting, diarrhea, rash, abnormal heart rhythm, jaundice due to elevated bilirubin	Should not be taken with Viagra, St. John's Wort; don't take antacids or drugs such as Prilosec, Protonix, or Nexium

Medication	Forms	Dose	How to take	Side Effects	Interactions
Viracept (nelfinavir)	250mg & 625mg tablets	(2) 625mg tablets twice daily; (5) 250mg tablets twice daily	Take with a snack or light meal	Most everyone will experience diarrhea	Should not be taken with Viagra, St. John's Wort

NON-NUCLEOSIDES (NNRTIS)

Medication	Forms	Dose	How to take	Side Effects	Interactions
Atripla (efavirenz + emtricitabine + tenofovir)	Tablets containing 600mg efavirenz, 200mg emtricitabine, 300mg tenofovir	(1) tablet at bedtime	Take on empty stomach	Vivid, life-like dreams, anxiety, difficulty concentrating, headache, nausea/ vomiting, rash. May exacerbate Hepatitis B. Can cause lactic acidosis characterized by fever, weakness, "sick feeling," muscle pain and weakness, fatigue. Elevated liver enzymes	Dose adjustments needed with Kaletra and Crixivan; *can't be taken during pregnancy.* Never take in regimen containing Truvada.
Viramune (neviripine)	200mg tablets	(2) tablets once daily or (1) tablet twice daily. Lead-in dosing of (1) tablet once daily for first two weeks of therapy	Take with or without food	Rash, headache, nausea, vomiting, diarrhea, fatigue, weakness, *severe liver toxicity*	May decrease effectiveness of oral contraceptives. Two forms of birth control should be used while taking Viramune.

Medication	Forms	Dose	How to take	Side Effects	Interactions
Rescriptor (delavirdine)	100mg and 200mg tablets	(2) 200mg tablets three times daily or (1) 600mg tablet twice daily	Take with or without food; take 1 hour apart from antacids	Nausea, vomiting, diarrhea, rash, elevated liver enzymes	Take 1 hour apart from antacids; dose adjustments may be needed when used with protease inhibitors
Sustiva (efavirenz)	200mg capsules and 600mg tablets	(3) 200mg capsules or (1) 600mg tablet at bedtime	Take on empty stomach a couple hours before bedtime	Vivid, life-like dreams, anxiety, difficulty concentrating, drowsiness, rash, symptoms of depression	Dose adjustments needed with Kaletra and Crixivan; *can't be taken during pregnancy*

NUCLEOTIDE ANALOGUE (A TYPE OF NRTI)

Medication	Forms	Dose	How to take	Side Effects	Interactions
Viread (tenofovir)	300mg tablet	(1) 300mg tablet once daily	Must be taken with food; take 1 hour before or 2 hours after Videx EC	Nausea, vomiting, diarrhea, elevated liver enzymes, changes in fat distribution	Dose adjustment and boosting of Reyataz if taken with Viread; Dose adjustment of Videx EC when taken with Viread

NUCLEOSIDES (NRTIS)

Medication	Forms	Dose	How to take	Side Effects	Interactions
Retrovir (zidovudine, AZT)	100mg capsule and 300mg tablet	(3) 100mg capsules or (1) 300mg tablet twice each day	May take with or without food — must have frequent blood counts done	Headache, fatigue, low blood counts— anemia characterized by fatigue, pale skin, weakness, shortness of breath	Dose adjustments in patients with renal disease and children. Should not be used with Zerit

Medication	Forms	Dose	How to take	Side Effects	Interactions
Combivir (retrovir + lamivudine)	Tablets containing 300mg retrovir and 150mg lamivudine	(1) tablet twice each day	May take with or without food — must have frequent blood counts done	Headache, fatigue, low blood counts—anemia characterized by fatigue, pale skin, weakness, shortness of breath	Should not be used with Zerit or the individual drugs lamivudine and retrovir.
Emtriva (emtricitabine)	200mg capsule	200mg once each day	Take with or without food	Headache, nausea/vomiting, rash. May exacerbate Hepatitis B. Can cause lactic acidosis characterized by fever, weakness, "sick feeling," muscle pain and weakness, fatigue	Never take in regimen containing Truvada
Epivir (lamivudine)	150mg and 300mg tablets	(1) 150mg tablet twice daily or (1) 300mg tablet once daily	Take with or without food	Headache, nausea, vomiting	Dose adjustments necessary in patients with renal disease
Epzicom (emtricitabine + abacavir)	Tablets containing 300mg lamivudine and 600mg abacavir	(1) tablet once each day	Take with or without food	Generalized sick feeling, flu-like symptoms, nausea, vomiting, rash, fatigue, headache, abdominal pain, dizziness	***Hypersensitivity reactions have been associated with Ziagen. Never stop and restart Ziagen or Ziagen-containing products—increased incidence of hypersensitivity results.***

Medication	Forms	Dose	How to take	Side Effects	Interactions
Hivid (zalcitabine)	0.75mg tablets	(1) tablet three times each day	Take with or without food	Numbness, tingling, burning of feet, hands, nausea, vomiting, rash, mouth ulcers, fever	Should not be taken with Videx EC (didanosine) or antacids
Trizivir (retrovir + lamivudine + abacavir)	Tablets containing 150mg lamivudine, 300mg retrovir, 300mg abacavir	(1) tablet twice each day	Take with or without food	Generalized sick feeling, flu-like symptoms, nausea, vomiting, rash, fatigue, headache, abdominal pain, dizziness	*Hypersensitivity reactions have been associated with Ziagen. Never stop and restart Ziagen or Ziagen-containing products—increased incidence of hypersensitivity results.*
Truvada (tenofovir + emtricitabine)	Tablets containing 200mg emtricitabine and 300mg tenofovir	(1) tablet once each day	Must be taken with food	Headaches, increased blood pressure, generalized "sick feeling," loss of appetite, rash, increase in liver enzymes	This class of drug has been associated with lactic acidosis. Not to be taken with the individual drugs Emtriva and Viread
Videx EC (didanosine)— Also available in generic form	200mg, 250mg and 400mg capsules	(1) capsule once each day	Take on an empty stomach 1 hour before or 2 hours after meals.	Abdominal pain, nausea, vomiting that may signal pancreatitis, burning in feet, hands, altered taste	Has been associated with lactic acidosis. Pentamidine increases the risk of pancreatitis
Zerit (stavudine)	15mg, 20mg, 30mg and 40mg capsules	80mg daily in one dose or divided doses	Take with or without food and 8oz of water	Numbness, tingling, burning in feet or hands, abdominal pain, nausea, vomiting	*This drug has been associated with lactic acidosis.*

Medication	Forms	Dose	How to take	Side Effects	Interactions
Ziagen (abacavir)	300mg tablets	(1) tablet twice each day	May take with or without food. ***Never stop and restart Ziagen.***	Generalized sick feeling, flu-like symptoms, nausea, vomiting, rash, fatigue, headache, abdominal pain, dizziness	*Hypersensitivity reactions have been associated with Ziagen. Never stop and restart Ziagen or Ziagen-containing products—increased incidence of hypersensitivity results.*

The Importance of Medication Adherence

The data is in, and as we have all heard, HIV medications have made HIV/AIDS a chronic disease much like asthma, diabetes or high blood pressure. Before the advent of medications, people were diagnosed only after symptoms of AIDS were exhibited. Without treatment options, infected people died soon after their diagnosis. Fortunately, that's not the case today. HIV testing and effective medications have forever changed the futures of those diagnosed. People are diagnosed sooner in the course of the illness, often very soon after the initial infection. Treatment options have made it possible to go on living after diagnosis. Simply put, medications have given HIV-infected people hope.

But just taking the medications is not enough. The effectiveness of HIV medications depends a great deal on how religiously they are taken. In other words, the medications will do their job of controlling the virus if they are taken everyday exactly as prescribed. HIV experts called such commitment to therapy *adherence*. Poor adherence is the number one reason medication regimens fail. But why is medication adherence such an integral part of a successful regimen? To answer that question let's look at one of the most important concepts in HIV care: *viral mutation and viral resistance.*

Viral Mutation

As discussed in an earlier chapter, HIV replicates (makes copies of itself) by using its own genetic material as well as the genetic material of its human host. In a perfect system, each HIV copy would be exactly like the last, from the coating on the outside of the virus particle to the genetic material within that particle. But in life, there is rarely a perfect system. HIV is no exception. While it's true that the majority of HIV copies are exactly like the one before, an occasional mistake occurs during replication. A small error is made during HIV replication, and that small error is then copied over and over, from new particle to new particle. Soon there are thousands of virus particles, each with the same small mistake. This natural process is called viral mutation. Let's look at a more practical example.

Imagine you have a document that needs to be copied for a big meeting. Using the office copy machine you begin making copies of the original document. After twenty identical copies, a small change occurs; in the case of our example, small dust particles cling to the original. These small particles cause each successive copy to have a black streak across the top of the page, obscuring most of the text. In this example dust particles have mutated our original, making it impossible to read. That mutation has been passed on to each subsequent copy. This example is a simple one, but it does illustrate how one small change can have a lasting impact, and how that change is carried from copy to copy.

How Do Mutations Occur?

We know what mutations are, but how do they occur in the first place? How does a normal, functioning virus particle mutate by itself? The answer is that it doesn't happen by itself. In our copy machine example, the dust particle that caused the black streak just didn't appear out of nowhere. Some environmental force acted upon the original, causing a mutation that was passed on with each copy. In this case a breeze in the copy room, or vibration from the machine deposited the dust particle that caused the mutation — the black streak on the paper.

Many environmental factors can cause mutations to occur in an HIV particle. The most important of those factors, ironically enough, is exposure to HIV medications. The same medications that prolong and improve the lives of HIV-infected people cause mutations that will eventually complicate HIV treatment. How can that happen?

Logic tells us that if HIV medications interfere with HIV replication then mutations shouldn't occur. In the presence of an effective therapy, very few HIV copies are being made; therefore there are fewer HIV copies to mutate. In a perfect system, that theory is a valid one. Mutations shouldn't occur or should occur at a less frequent rate when the medications are taken as prescribed. The key is to take the medications as prescribed — in other words, to adhere to the HIV medication regimen.

What Is Medication Adherence?

Steadman's Medical Dictionary defines adherence as *the extent to which the patient continues the agreed-upon mode of treatment under limited supervision when faced with conflicting demands.* Simply put, adherence refers to the patient's willingness to take his or her medicines as prescribed each and every day, despite the daily demands of living with HIV. If a patient is able to adhere, then the medications will do their job and keep the virus from replicating. Without replication, there is no mutation. In turn, if the medications are taken inconsistently or sporadically, the virus is allowed to replicate, which will result in a mutated virus.

So How Do Mutations Affect the HIV Patient?

So we know what mutations are, and we know how they occur. We also know how medication adherence affects the development of mutations. But how does all this impact the HIV-infected person?

Remember, mutations are changes in the genetic structure of the HIV particle. HIV medications are designed with a certain HIV genetic structure in mind. Consequently, medications are effective against HIV particles that have typical genetic structures— in other words, mutation free. Mutations alter the genetic structure, making medications less effective in slowing HIV replication. As more and more mutated viral copies are made, the medicines become less and less effective, eventually becoming unable to slow replication at all. With the right mutations, HIV is able to resist the very medications used to slow their replication. This concept is known as *resistance.*

HIV Resistance

Resistance is just that — HIV's ability to resist or be resistant to the beneficial effects of HIV medications normally able to control the virus. Poor medication adherence leads to viral resistant. Once resistant, HIV is able to replicate freely, despite the presence of medications.

Let's go back to our copy machine example. The manufacturer of the copy machine recommends regular cleaning with a special solvent to minimize and eliminate dust that could cause poor copies. If the user follows this recommendation, dust will not accumulate, and each copy will be perfect. In this example, the cleaning solvent represents HIV medications, and using the solvent as prescribed by the manufacturer represents medication adherence. Adhere to the manufacturer's "prescription" and each copy will be perfect.

However, if the user ignores the maintenance recommendations of the manufacturer, dust will accumulate and poor copy quality will result. In other words, the accumulated dust will cause mutated copies. Once the mutated copies have occurred, cleaning with the solvent will not improve the quality of future copies. The damage has been done. While this comparison may be a stretch, understand that without medication adherence, mutations will occur and the medications will inevitably become less effective.

Resistance to individual medications is just the tip of the iceberg. When resistance to a current medication occurs, that resistance will often translate to all of the drugs in that class. For instance, if resistance develops to a specific NNRTI, it's possible that resistance will translate to all of the NNRTIs, even the NNRTIs that the person has never taken. This severely limits choices for future regimens, making treatment much more difficult and often impossible. Like dust on the copy, medication resistance has a far-reaching impact.

Why Do People Have Poor Adherence?

As our extensive discussion of viral mutation and resistance has illustrated, improving medication adherence improves therapy effectiveness as well. HIV medical professionals and educators alike constantly reinforce the importance of adherence as part of their medical practices, through patient education programs, and by providing adherence tools to their patients. So why do people still have difficulty adhering to the very medications that could improve and extend their lives?

Common sense tells us that with such overwhelming evidence that adherence is important, people would gladly take their medicines exactly as prescribed. Yet, poor adherence continues to be the biggest problem surrounding HIV treatment. The fact is that adherence to HIV medications is not an easy proposition, despite its well known benefits and a person's commitment to taking medications. There are several factors that interfere with drug adherence. Let's take a look at the most common.

- *State of Mind:* It became obvious soon after the epidemic emerged that HIV affects far more than just the physical self. In fact, the emotional self is affected as much as, or in many cases, more than the physical self. Feelings of guilt, anger, depression, and isolation are just some of the emotional issues HIV-infected people deal with on a day to day basis. These emotional issues make medication adherence extremely difficult, especially if there are unpleasant side effects from the medications. Before a person can adhere to medications, his or her emotional issues surrounding their diagnosis must be dealt with.
- *Medication Side Effects:* Medication side effects are not unique to HIV drugs. Most prescription medications have some type of side effect, some more

severe and unpleasant than others. When HIV medications first emerged, they were notorious for their severe side effects. As the years passed, HIV drug manufacturers improved their medicines, diminishing side effects and creating new formulations of existing meds that have made them more palatable and easier to take. Yet, even with the significant improvements that have been made, side effects continue to make adhering to regimens difficult. Many people report feeling worse on medications then they do off medications. Imagine adhering to medications that physically make you feel worse than how you felt before starting them. How do health care providers convince people that the medications that are making them nauseated, tired, and weak are the same medications that will help them live longer? That's the key to adherence teaching, and it's not easy.

• *Cost of Medications:* It's no secret that HIV medications are very expensive. For those people without insurance or drug coverage, adhering to medication regimens is severely complicated by their cost. Even people with insurance and drug coverage may have difficulty paying the deductibles required by their insurer. If a person can't afford deductibles or the price of medications, adherence is impossible.

• *Complexity of Regimens:* Taking one medication can be difficult. Taking a regimen of three or four HIV medications, along with preventative antibiotics, can be impossible for many people. There are medications that need to be taken on an empty stomach, others need to be taken with food, and still others need to taken separate from the other medications in the regimen. The more complex the drug regimen the less likely the regimen will be adhered to.

• *Patient Limitations:* People living with HIV may have characteristics and traits that can make adherence difficult. Busy lifestyles, work schedules, and school schedules can complicate medication adherence. Social obstacles, such as the inability to read, a poor understanding of the English language, or being homeless, also contribute to poor adherence. Perhaps the best predictor of adherence is a person's desire, willingness, or commitment to take HIV medications. Without a true commitment to medications, adherence is literally impossible.

Tips to Improve Adherence

We have established the importance of medication adherence. But what can be done to improve the ability of HIV infected people to take their medications as prescribed? There are a number of ways to improve HIV medication adherence. Not all of them will work for everyone. The key is to find what works for you.

- *Combat the Hectic Schedule:* One common obstacle to medication adherence is a busy schedule that interferes with medication adherence. There are ways to improve adherence even for those people with hectic schedules.
  - Set up medications ahead of time using pill boxes. These important tools of adherence are usually available free of charge from your doctor's office. They can also be purchased at most retail pharmacies or online. Depending on your regimen and the number of pills you take each day, pill boxes can be set up a week ahead of time, saving time and assuring that each day you have the proper pills in the proper doses ready to take with the least amount of effort.
  - Pill boxes are comprised of seven individual day compartments that can be removed and carried in a pocket, lunch box, or brief case. This saves time and improves adherence by keeping your pills close at hand wherever you go.
  - People often get busy or lose track of time, causing them to miss a dose or doses of their medication. Wearing a watch or a medication timer with an alarm will help minimize or eliminate missed doses by notifying the wearer when it's time to take his or her medicine. Many companies or pharmacies sell medication alarms. For those unable to afford alarms, many HIV agencies or medical practices will provide them for their patients or will help find resources to purchase one.

- *Confidentiality:* Many fear that taking medications while at work or school will "tip off" their friends or coworkers to their HIV diagnosis. People choose to miss doses rather than risk jeopardizing their confidentiality by taking medications in a place where others may see them. To maintain confidentiality while taking all your doses, carry medications in a small pill box. When it is time for medications to be taken, excuse yourself to the restroom or step outside for a break. This allows you to take your medicine each and every day while maintaining your confidentiality. If you are seen taking medicines, remember you are not obligated to share your medical information with anyone; your confidentiality is protected by law.

- *We Are All Forgetful:* Being human, we all forget things—including when to take our medicine. People who are dealing with opportunistic infections may have poor short-term and long-term memory. Leave notes around your home, in places where you will be sure to see them — the refrigerator, the television or the bathroom medicine cabinet or mirror. Leave your pill bottles or pill boxes in places you will be sure to find them — the kitchen sink, next to your toothbrush, or with your car keys. If you have a friend or loved one who is aware of your diagnosis, ask them to help you remember by calling you when it is time for your pills. Finally, in many communities there are "buddy programs" that bring together people who are HIV-infected to remind each other and to offer support for one another when adherence is a problem.

• *Not Sure Where the Problem Lies:* For some people it's hard to identify problems with adherence until the medication regimen has been started. In fact, it's hard to predict exactly who will have adherence problems and who won't. There are ways, however, to identify adherence issues before starting your medicines. Take a trial run of your regimen using jelly beans, a different color for each type of medicine. Take the jelly beans as you would your medicines. Fine tune your medication schedule until you find one that results in the best adherence and fewest missed or forgotten doses. If jelly-bean doses are missed, make a note of the reason and remedy it before starting your medications for real. Identifying problems before starting your medications will improve your chances of adherence without the risk of mutation and resistance.

The Problem of Medication Side Effects

The biggest obstacles to medication adherence are the side effects inherent to each HIV medication. While the side effect profiles of HIV medications have improved dramatically in the last ten years, side effects are still a reality and must be dealt with by most people to some degree or another. While some HIV medications have side effects that resolve over time, others have untoward affects that last as long as the person is taking the drugs. Let's look at the most common side effects and what can be done to resolve them.

NAUSEA

Probably the most common of all side effects, nausea is associated with several HIV medications. Some of the biggest culprits are Norvir (ritonavir) and Kaletra (lopinavir + ritonavir). Most nausea occurs when the therapy is started but resolves a few weeks later. Nausea can also occur when certain medications are taken on an empty stomach. There are ways to combat nausea that does not resolve on its own.

• Change your diet, first to clear liquids, then add bland foods as you can tolerate. A BRAT diet is one that is comprised of bananas, rice, applesauce and toast — easy to digest foods that give the stomach time to recover. Introduce each of these four foods one at a time, giving the intestinal tract and stomach time to "rest," helping the body resolve the nausea. As the nausea decreases, add more complex foods as tolerated.

• Leave dry crackers at your bedside. Each morning before getting out of bed, eat a few crackers and rest for a few minutes. This method is widely used by pregnant women to relieve the nausea of morning sickness.

- When nausea strikes, drink cool, carbonated liquids such as ginger ale or clear soda pops. Pharmacies sometime stock Coca Cola syrup (Coke syrup without the carbonated water) that can be taken in small amounts to ease nausea. The Coke syrup is usually stocked behind the pharmacy counter, so ask your pharmacist.
- If the nausea is not relieved by the simple remedies above, your doctor can prescribe medications that will help. There are downsides to this solution, however. A prescription to combat nausea means at least one more pill to take each day. There is also a chance of unpleasant side effects from the anti-nausea medication, such as anxiety and restlessness.
- Many times, resolving nausea associated with HIV medications is just a matter of taking them with food. Just make note of your regimen and what medications can and can't be taken with food. Ask your doctor or your pharmacist which medication can be taken with food.
- Often, vomiting will accompany nausea. If this occurs, use the same remedies as you would to combat nausea, but concentrate on increasing the amount of fluids you drink each day. While carbonated beverages help with nausea, once vomiting begins, plain cool water or electrolyte replacement drinks like Gatorade or Pedialyte are best to prevent the dehydration that results from serious or long-term vomiting. How do you know you are dehydrated? Symptoms include:
  - headache
  - dizziness, especially when changing position
  - lightheadedness
  - dry skin, lips, tongue or mucous membranes
  - decreased elasticity of the skin
  - rapid heart rate (greater than 100 beats per minute)

If you are unable to keep hydrated by increasing your fluid intake, seek medical care immediately. Very often a more invasive means of fluid replacement, such as intravenous fluids, may be needed to reverse your dehydration.

DIARRHEA

Undoubtedly the most inconvenient and uncomfortable side effect of HIV medications is diarrhea. While many HIV medications can cause diarrhea, the most notable is Viracept (nelfinavir). As is the case with vomiting, diarrhea can cause dehydration, therefore, those steps discussed earlier should be implemented to prevent dehydration. There are several ways to resolve diarrhea. They include:

- Eating foods high in *soluble fiber*—fiber that attracts water — including oatmeal, breads, and wheat products. Dietary fiber is not digestible by the human intestinal tract, but it does slow digestion, which in turn increases absorption. High soluble fiber foods help slow diarrhea by absorbing excess water normally absorbed in the intestinal tract.

- Avoid foods that have *insoluble fiber*—fiber that does not dissolve in water—such as fruit and vegetable skin. Insoluble fiber holds water that will make the stool moist and loose. Obviously when diarrhea strikes, extra intestinal water is the last thing needed.
- Avoid greasy or spicy foods, as well as dairy products, all of which can aggravate diarrhea.
- As is the case with vomiting, diarrhea can cause dehydration. Fluids must be replaced as quickly as they are lost to prevent dehydration. Increasing the intake of such fluids as water or electrolyte sports drinks will most likely not improve diarrhea, but it will prevent the dehydration that results.

DRY MOUTH

Many medications used to control HIV and prevent opportunistic infections can cause dry mouth. However, dry mouth can be combated in several ways. They include:

- Rinse your mouth with warm salt water several times per day. However, caution must be taken to avoid water that is too salty, which can actually worsen dry mouth.
- Hard candy and lozenges used throughout the day can alleviate dry mouth. For those people living with diabetes, make sure the candies are sugar free so the blood sugar is not negatively affected.
- In extreme cases of dry mouth, your doctor can prescribe medicines that will replace the mouth's natural moisture. If mouth pain occurs, or breaks in the mucous membranes of the mouth or tongue are present, notify your doctor immediately.

FATIGUE

A few HIV medications can cause feelings of fatigue or a lack of energy. Fatigue can simply be the result of HIV, similar to the fatigue one gets when suffering from the flu virus, for example. When fatigue is caused by medications, there are ways to diminish the symptoms. They include:

- First and foremost, the body needs adequate rest and exercise. When you are fatigued you may sleep most of the day. However, this doesn't mean you are getting enough quality sleep. Eight hours of uninterrupted sleep each night is the best way to feel rested and energetic.
- When energy levels are low, as is the case with fatigue, summoning the energy to exercise is very difficult. But by increasing your level of exercise you can increase your energy level and relieve the symptoms of fatigue.

- Follow a healthy diet, one rich in vitamins, minerals and representing all the food groups. Many HIV medical practices have a nutritionist on staff or can refer you to one in order to help you put together a healthy diet that will improve your symptoms of fatigue.
- If you suffer from fatigue, never assume that it is being caused by the medications you are taking. Conditions such as depression, low hormone levels, or a low blood count (anemia) can cause fatigue as well. In order to treat your fatigue, the doctor must determine the cause. If you suffer from fatigue, notify your doctor immediately.

Rash / Itching

Rashes with and without itching skin can have many causes, including liver disease, allergies, foods, and certain medications. If you develop a rash with or without itching you should notify your doctor immediately. While you are waiting to see your doctor, there are measures you can take relieve your symptoms. They include:

- Avoid hot baths or showers, which could aggravate rashes. When showering or bathing, use warm or tepid water and do not stay in the water longer than necessary.
- Direct sunlight can cause or aggravate a rash. In fact, Bactrim, an antibiotic used to prevent and treat pneumocystis pneumonia, makes the skin much more sensitive to sunlight and can cause or worsen a rash. If you take Bactrim or another medication that can increase your risk of a rash, sunlight must be avoided.
- Liver disease can cause generalized itching. For this reason, any time you experience itching, you should notify your doctor immediately. A simple blood test can tell your doctor if your itching is related to an undiagnosed liver disease.
- Before stopping any medications due to a rash, consult your doctor first. The HIV medication Ziagen (abacavir), and any medication containing abacavir, can't be stopped and restarted. Doing so can increase the risk of the severe allergic reaction (hypersensitivity reaction) sometimes experienced by people taking abacavir.

Depression

Along with the emotional causes of depression, there is one specific HIV medication that can cause or exacerbate the symptoms of depression. Sustiva (efavirenz) has been known to cause depression in those people not previously depressed, and to worsen symptoms in those people with an existing diagnosis of depression. Unlike the side effects discussed earlier, depression is one that should not be addressed by the patient alone. Instead, when symptoms of depression do arise, a remedy should be left to professionals—your HIV specialist, a psychiatrist or a psychologist. If symptoms occur, notify your doctor as soon as possible.

The one thing patients can do to combat depression is to be alert for its signs and symptoms. Know your body and recognize when you are not feeling what's normal for you. Because depression is such an important and complex issue, we will discuss how to recognize the signs and symptoms in a later chapter.

This chapter has taught us that HIV medications have been the key to longer, healthier lives since their introduction over a decade ago. We have also illustrated the importance of adhering to your prescribed medication regimen, and the negative impact viral mutations and resistance can have on your health. Unfortunately, like any chronic illness, HIV will rear its ugly head now and again. What happens when HIV eventually chips away at your natural defenses? In the next chapter we will discuss opportunistic infections common to HIV, how to recognize them before they make you sick, and how to prevent and treat them.

8

Opportunistic Infections

The purpose of HIV medications, of all the doctors and nurses who care for HIV patients, of all things related to HIV healthcare, even the purpose of this book is to help people living with HIV stay healthy as long as possible. Obviously, HIV can be very detrimental to the immune system of those people infected with the virus. As the immune system becomes damaged from HIV, the body becomes at risk for certain infections and illnesses. This chapter deals with those illnesses and infections that jeopardize the health of every person living with HIV. We will look at the collection of infections that are common in HIV, learn how to recognize the signs and symptoms of those infections, and, finally, learn how to prevent them from occurring in the first place.

The Big Myth — HIV Makes You Sick

There are many myths and misconceptions surrounding HIV and AIDS, not the least of which is the belief that HIV makes a person sick. I may be exaggerating when I say this, but nothing could be farther from the truth. We all know that millions have died after becoming infected with HIV, but the truth is that HIV did not make all those people sick. Let's explain what I mean.

Earlier in this text we discussed the affects of HIV on the human body. For the sake of review, HIV uses the body's immune system to make copies of itself. Specifically, HIV uses CD4 cells to replicate, or, in other words, to make copies of itself. Unfortunately, CD4 cells are damaged in the process. The more CD4 cells that are damaged, the weaker our immune system becomes— eventually becoming so weak that the immune system is unable to protect the body from infection and illness. So you see, it's not HIV that makes a person sick, it's the weakened immune system that results in illness and infection. HIV does the damage to the immune system, but it's the infections and illnesses that arise because of the weakened immune system that makes the HIV-infected person sick. Is this just a matter of semantics? Possibly, but the concept is an important one. If indeed HIV does damage the immune system, then logic says that the key to keeping the HIV-infected person healthy is to limit immune system damage and prevent those infections that take advantage of the weakened immune system. Or, in other words, the key is to prevent opportunistic infections.

Opportunistic Infections

Exactly as the name implies, opportunistic infections exploit the opportunity to make a person sick when the immune system is at its weakest. Most opportunistic infections are caused by organisms that are essentially harmless in the presence of a healthy immune system. For example, most every adult has been exposed to the cytomegalovirus (CMV) some time in their life. The majority of these people have a normal immune system which prevents CMV from doing any harm. But in people with a weakened immune system, such as the HIV-infected person, CMV can wreak havoc, causing serious infections throughout the body.

Opportunistic infections are caused by many organisms, including bacteria, viruses, parasites, and fungi. Let's look at these organisms and the most common infections they cause.

BACTERIAL

Mycobacterium Avium Complex (MAC)

MAC is a bacterial infection transferred from person to person primarily via the water supply. However, there is really no good way to prevent exposure. In the normal functioning immune system, MAC can exist in the body without doing harm. But in the weakened immune system, MAC can cause serious infections. Usually MAC starts in the intestinal tract.

- Symptoms — Night sweats, weight loss, abdominal pain, diarrhea with blood and/or white blood cells in stool, elevated liver enzymes (especially alkaline phosphatase).
- Risk Level — People are at greater risk when the CD4 count is 50 cells/mm^3 or less. Prophylaxis medications begin when the CD4 falls below 100 cells/mm^3.
- Prevention/Prophylaxis — The drugs azithromycin, rifabutin, or clarithromycin are started when the CD4 count falls below 100 cells/mm^3.
- Treatment — Several antibiotics, including azithromycin, rifabutin, clarithromycin, ethambutol, or ciprofloxacin, are used to treat MAC infection.

Tuberculosis (TB)

Decades ago, TB was a serious illness found throughout the world. But with effective medications it was all but eliminated in the western world. However, with the emergence of HIV, TB has once again become a serious problem. Many people are infected with TB early in life, but it remains inactive and they remain symptom free. However, many people's TB activates when their immune system becomes too weak to protect them any longer. More disturbing yet is the emergence of a resistant type of TB—a strain resistant to the antibiotics that are typically an effective treatment. TB is highly contagious, spread from person to person by water droplets released into the air when coughing or sneezing. TB most commonly affects the lungs (pulmonary) but can infect other parts of the body (extrapulmonary) as well. TB can be active (infectious, and making a person sick) or latent (non-contagious and without symptoms of illness).

- Symptoms—Fatigue, night sweats, a cough producing blood-tinged sputum, fever, weight loss.
- Risk Level—While active TB usually strikes those people with CD4 counts less than 200cells/mm^3, it can activate and become infectious at any CD4 count.
- Prevention/Prophylaxis—The drug isoniazid is used to prevent latent TB from becoming active.
- Treatment—Usually a multiple drug regimen that can include isoniazid, rifampin, pyrazinamide, ethambutol or streptomycin. With resistant strains of TB, susceptibility tests must be done to see which antibiotic will be effective.

TABLE 8. TYPES OF TUBERCULOSIS

Active
- Typically strikes people with weakened immune systems, including those with HIV.
- Symptoms include fatigue; night sweats; cough producing blood tinged sputum; fever; and weight loss.
- Effectively treated with multiple drug regimens.

Inactive
- TB-infected, but no signs or symptoms of illness.
- Typically will not activate unless the immune system becomes weakened for some reason.
- Medications are prescribed to prevent the TB from becoming active.

Salmonellosis ("food poisoning")

This bacterial infection is spread by way of contaminated food or water, thus the name "food poisoning." The risk of becoming infected with salmonella increases when raw meats or eggs are ingested. Therefore it is important to cook those foods thoroughly before eating. Because salmonella can be found in feces, the spread of salmonella from person to person is also possible through oral to anal contact.

- Symptoms—Abdominal pain, severe diarrhea, bloody stools, chills, a loss of appetite beginning one to three days after exposure.

- Risk Level — Salmonella can infect people with any CD4 count but is more common in people infected with HIV.
- Prevention/Prophylaxis— The best way to prevent salmonella is by frequent, proper hand washing, especially after using the bathroom or after handling raw meats, poultry and eggs. People with HIV should avoid foods that contain raw eggs, such as chocolate mousse, caesar salad dressing, and raw cake and cookie batter. Poultry products, such as chicken and turkey, should be cooked thoroughly before eating. Steaks and pork should not be served rare. After preparing foods, kitchen counters and cutting boards should be cleaned with bleach and disposable wash cloths. Make sure certain foods are refrigerator prior to cooking, and that leftovers are refrigerated promptly after the meal.
- Treatment — Antibiotics, such as ciprofloxacin, Bactrim, chloramphenicol, and ampicillin, are used to treat infection.

Syphilis

This sexually transmitted infection is caused by a worm-like bacterium called a *spirochete*. The genus and species name for this spirochete is *Treponema pallidum*. There are three stages to syphilis, each exhibiting different symptoms.

- Symptoms—*Primary infection* is characterized by painless lesions on the genitals. These lesions will heal after a few weeks, but the bacterium that caused the syphilis does not heal; there is no cure. *Secondary syphilis* is characterized by a rash and fever. *Latent syphilis* can cause lesions on internal organs such as the brain and central nervous system. Left untreated, latent syphilis can be fatal.
- Risk Level — Syphilis can strike anyone regardless of their CD4 count.
- Prevention/Prophylaxis— The only way to prevent a syphilis infection is to use a latex condom during all anal, oral, or vaginal sexual encounters.
- Treatment — The first treatment choice is a series of three penicillin injections, each one week apart. For those allergic to penicillin, the antibiotics doxycycline and ceftriaxone can be used.

TABLE 9. THE STAGES OF SYPHILIS

Primary Infection
- Painless lesions on the genitals.
- The lesions heal but the bacterium remains.

Secondary Syphilis
- Characterized by rash and fever.

Latent Syphilis
- Can cause lesions on internal organs such as the brain and other parts of the central nervous system.
- Left untreated, latent syphilis can be fatal.

Bacillary Angiomatosis ("cat scratch disease")

This bacterial infection is associated with cat scratch disease, an infection caused by cat fleas. *Bacillary angiomatosis* is extremely rare in people who aren't infected with HIV. Often it's confused with Kaposi's sarcoma due to similarities in appearance. Bacillary angiomatosis is related to an infection called *trench fever*, common among soldiers in World War I. Left untreated, bacillary angiomatosis can be fatal.

- Symptoms— This infection is characterized by nodules or lesions on and just below the surface of the skin. As the number of nodules increase, patients may develop fever, chills, poor appetite, weight loss, and night sweats. The infection can also spread to the bone and bone marrow, spleen, liver, and lymph nodes. These bacteria can also cause blood vessels to grow out of control, resulting in purplish lesions that closely resemble the lesions of Kaposi's sarcoma.

- Risk Level— Bacillary angiomatosis is found almost exclusively in patients infected with HIV, most frequently in those people with CD4 counts less than 500cells/mm^3. Obviously, exposure to cats and cat fleas dramatically increases the risk of acquiring this disease.

- Prevention/Prophylaxis— Avoid cats and cat fleas.

- Treatment— As potentially serious as the infection is, it is easily treated with several weeks of doxycycline and erythromycin.

Bacterial Pneumonia

A bacterial infection that causes irritation, swelling, and congestion in the lungs. This bacterial infection usually follows a cold. It is also known as *pneumonitis*.

- Symptoms— The onset of symptoms is usually sudden. They include fever, chills, difficulty breathing, a cough producing bloody or yellow sputum, fatigue, feeling tired, blue or pale lips or nail beds.

- Risk Level— Studies have shown that bacterial pneumonia can occur with any CD4 count but does occur more frequently in patients with HIV. The severity of the bacterial pneumonia is also greater in people with HIV.

- Prevention/Prophylaxis— There are vaccines available that help decrease the risk of bacterial pneumonia. Evidence suggests that Bactrim taken once each day can decrease the risk of bacterial pneumonia. Finally, people taking HIV-medications have a lower incidence of bacterial pneumonia than do HIV positive patients not on HIV medications.

- Treatment— Antibiotic therapy is the treatment of choice for bacterial pneumonia. The type of antibiotic depends on the type of bacteria causing the pneumonia.

Fungal

Pneumocystis Carinii Pneumonia (PCP) / Pneumocystis Jiroveci Pneumonia

At one time experts thought PCP was caused by a parasite. Actually, PCP is caused by a yeast-like fungus called *Pneumocystis jiroveci.* The fungus typically infects the lungs of people with weakened immune systems. At the outset of the HIV epidemic it was PCP infection that first brought people to the emergency department. Even today, for many people the first symptom of HIV is a diagnosis of PCP. Unfortunately, by the time PCP occurs there has already been significant damage done to the immune system. Before the use of prophylaxis antibiotics such as Bactrim, PCP was common and often fatal among HIV-infected people. It was an unusually high incidence of new PCP cases in the early 1980s that signaled the beginning of the HIV epidemic.

- Symptoms—PCP causes shortness of breath, a dry cough, and difficulty breathing. Often, breathing difficulties are only evident after mild exertion such as walking. Fever is also present. As the infection progresses, the respiratory symptoms get worse, many times leading to hospitalization and the need for assisted breathing using a ventilator. If left untreated, PCP is fatal.
- Risk Level—PCP rarely occurs in people with CD4 counts greater than 200cells/mm^3.
- Prevention/Prophylaxis—The risk of acquiring PCP can be diminished with the use of prophylaxis antibiotics such as Bactrim, Pentamidine, Dapsone, and Atovaquone.
- Treatment—PCP is treated with the same antibiotics used to prevent the infection. However, higher doses and/or intravenous forms of the antibiotics are necessary. In addition, steroid therapy can be used to decrease inflammation caused by the PCP infection.

Aspergillosis

This type of fungus is most often found in soil and decaying plant life. Most often, the fungus is inhaled through the mouth and/or nose, primarily infecting the lungs or sinuses. Aspergillos is rare, most often striking those people with significantly compromised immune systems. In addition to HIV patients with significant immune system damage, other populations at risk for Aspergillos include cancer patients undergoing chemotherapy and transplant patients on anti-rejection medications.

- Symptoms—The symptoms of Aspergillos are similar to those found in lung or sinus infections. If the primary site of infection is the lungs, symptoms will include cough, chest pain, shortness of breath, and fever. An Aspergillos infection of the sinuses will cause headache, facial pain and fever. Night sweats can characterize any Aspergillos infection.

- Risk Level — Most people who develop an Aspergillos infection have a CD4 count of less than 100 cells/mm^3. However, infection can occur in people with CD4 counts greater than 100 cells/mm^3 under certain circumstances. People living with AIDS (having a CD4 count less than 200 cells/mm^3) often develop Aspergillos after suffering from bacterial or pneumocystis pneumonia.
- Prevention / Prophylaxis — There is no specific prophylaxis used to prevent Aspergillos. Instead, taking precautions when handling soil or plant life during yard work is suggested. Those at particularly high risk should wear gloves and masks when gardening or working outside. Good hand washing is also suggested.
- Treatment — Very potent antifungal medications must be used to treat Aspergillos. Oral intraconazole and intravenous amphotericin B are the treatments of choice.

Candidiasis ("thrush," "candida," "yeast infection")

The most common fungal infection, candidiasis is caused by the fungus *Candida albicans,* one of many species of candida fungi. Candidiasis occurs in the moist mucous membranes of the mouth, esophagus and vagina. On occasion, candidiasis can occur on the skin.

- Symptoms — Candida infections of the mouth ("thrush") are characterized by white patches on the tongue, gums, roof of the mouth and the inside of the cheeks. These patches can cause altered taste, dry mouth, mouth soreness, and difficulty swallowing. Fungal infections of the esophagus ("candida esophagitis") cause chest pain, sore throat and, in extreme cases, difficulty swallowing and breathing. Finally, vaginal candida infections ("yeast infection") are characterized by vaginal itching, milky vaginal discharge, and vaginal irritation and/or pain.
- Risk Level — While anyone can have thrush regardless of CD4 count, the incidence increases when the CD4 count drops below 200 cells/mm^3.
- Prevention/Prophylaxis — Typically, prophylaxis medications are not prescribed to prevent thrush. In fact, there is not much data to support thrush prophylaxis. If prophylaxis is ordered, antifungal medications such as fluconazole are prescribed to be taken once per day. To prevent vaginal yeast infections, doctors suggest eating yogurt with active bacterial cultures. These bacteria help protect the vaginal area from infection.
- Treatment — Treatment for oral thrush, candida esophagitis, or vaginal yeast infections is in the form of antifungal medications. Fluconazole once per day, ranging from one day to two weeks or more, is common. Depending on the dose, yeast infections can be treated with as little as one dose of antifungal medication. For those not wanting to take oral medications, antifungal topical creams can be used to treat vaginal yeast infections; how-

ever, the incidence of reoccurrence is high. Finally, mild cases of oral candida can be treated with antifungal lozenges; however, they must be taken several times each day to be effective. As is the case with topical creams, the reoccurrence rate of candida after using antifungal lozenges is high.

Coccidioidomycosis

A fungus found primarily in soil throughout the Southwestern United States, Mexico, Central America, and South America. As part of its life cycle, the fungus becomes airborne. It's at this time that the fungus is most infectious, entering the body during inspiration and infecting the lungs. The lungs aren't the only organs that can be infected. Coccidioidomycosis infection can also involve the kidneys, lymph system, spleen and brain.

- Symptoms— Early symptoms include cough, weight loss and fatigue. If left untreated, the infection can spread to the brain and other parts of the central nervous system, causing headache, confusion, light sensitivity and fever. Without treatment, the infection will progress throughout the body, eventually resulting in death.
- Risk Level — The primary risk of coccidioidomycosis occurs once the CD4 count drops below 100 cells/mm^3. Keep in mind that the lowest CD4 point since HIV diagnosis should be the value used to assess the risk for coccidioidmycosis. For instance, if the current CD4 value is 250 cells/mm^3, but the CD4 count has been as low as 25 cells/mm^3 since diagnosis, the risk for coccidioidmycosis should be based on the lowest value since diagnosis of HIV — in this case, 25 cells/mm^3.
- Prevention/Prophylaxis— Precautions such as wearing gloves and a mask while working with soil should be employed. Currently, there is no medication that is used as a prophylaxis against coccidioidmycosis.
- Treatment — Antifungal medications are used to treat this fungal infection — oral fluconazole for mild cases and intravenous amphotericin B for more extensive and severe infections.

Cryptococcus

This yeast-like fungus is found in soil all over the world. *Cryptococcus neoformans* is found most commonly in soil contaminated with bird droppings. This fungus affects primarily the lungs and brain, but in advanced cases can affect other organs and cause lesions on the skin. Infection occurs when the fungus is inhaled into the lungs in the form of dehydrated spores. After lying dormant in the lungs, the fungus spreads to other tissues and organs, especially the lungs and brain. A cryptococcal infection in the brain (cryptococcal meningitis) is often fatal if left untreated, especially in people with severely weakened immune systems. In the lungs, this fungus causes cryptococcal pneumonia, a serious and potentially fatal respiratory infection.

- Symptoms—The symptoms of cryptococcus infection depend on the organs involved. Left untreated, symptoms worsen over the course of a few weeks. Cryptococcal meningitis symptoms include headache, fever, stiff neck, and sensitivity to light ("photophobia"). As the meningitis progresses, symptoms of brain swelling, such as nausea, vomiting, confusion, paralysis, and coma, emerge. Left untreated, a person can progress from coma to death in a short period of time. Cryptococcal pneumonia symptoms are much like those of bacterial pneumonia and pneumocystis pneumonia. These symptoms include fever, cough, shortness of breath, chest tightness and chest pain.

- Risk Level—The greatest risk of cryptococcus infection occurs once the CD4 count falls below 100 cells/mm^3. It's important to note that even in HIV-positive people whose CD4 counts have risen above 100 cells/mm^3, there is still a risk. To accurately assess the risk of cryptococcus infection, the lowest CD4 count since being diagnosed (nadir) with HIV should be used, regardless of how early in the course of the disease it was.

- Prevention/Prophylaxis—Taking precautions, such as wearing gloves and a mask while working with soil or birds, is the best way to reduce the risk of infection. Wearing a mask and gloves minimizes the risk of inhaling the fungal spores that cause infection. The antifungal medication *fluconazole* is sometimes used when the CD4 count drops below 100 cells/mm^3. Many practitioners are reluctant to use prophylaxis because of medication cost and the possibility that drug-resistant cryptococcal meningitis will develop. Drug resistant meningitis can be particularly serious because it does not respond to conventional anti-fungal treatment.

- Treatment—Oral medications such as the anti-fungal fluconazole can be used in less severe cases. In advanced cases of cryptococcal meningitis or pneumonia, intravenous amphotericin B can be used. Keep in mind that in people with severely weakened immune systems, treatment is often unsuccessful.

Histoplasmosis

An infection caused by the fungus *Histoplasma capsulatum*. This fungus is found in soil contaminated by bird droppings. Infection occurs when dehydrated spores are inhaled while working with contaminated soil or while cleaning a bird cage contaminated with infected bird droppings.

- Symptoms—The symptoms of histoplasmosis depend on the tissues and organs infected. Most often histoplasmosis affects the lungs, resulting in fever, difficulty breathing, shortness of breath and cough. If the infection progresses to organs other than the lungs it is said to be a *disseminated infection*—an infection throughout the body—and can cause skin lesions, weight loss, and an enlarged liver, spleen or lymph nodes. If histoplasmosis affects the bone marrow, platelet, white blood cell, and red blood cell production is compromised, resulting in low levels of these blood cell components.

- Risk Level — The risk of histoplasmosis increases when the CD4 count falls below 100 cells/mm^3. As in other types of fungal infections, the lowest known CD4 count since HIV diagnosis should be used to determine histoplasmosis infection risk.
- Prevention/Prophylaxis— The use of anti-fungals such as fluconazole is not recommended in people with healthy immune systems. However, prophylaxis may be done using fluconazole or the drug itraconazole for those people with CD4 counts below 100 cells/mm^3. Precautions such as wearing a mask and gloves while handling contaminated soil will limit exposure to the histoplasma, thus decreasing the risk of infection.
- Treatment — Treatment of histoplasmosis is a two step process— treatment for the acute infection and maintenance therapy after the acute infection has been resolved to prevent infection from recurring. Mild to moderate acute infection is treated with the oral drug *itraconazole*. For more severe infections, intravenous *amphotericin B* is required. Intravenous amphotericin B requires hospitalization and unfortunately can be very toxic to the kidneys and bone marrow. Because of this, close monitoring of kidney function and blood count is necessary. After the acute infection is treated, maintenance therapy must be initiated. In the case of those people with very weak immune systems, this maintenance therapy is often continued for life. Oral itraconazole is the primary maintenance drug, but in those people who have difficulty maintaining high enough itraconazole blood levels to prevent reoccurrence, oral fluconazole can be added.

VIRAL

Cytomegalovirus (CMV)

CMV is a virus from the group of viruses known as *herpesviridae*. There are eight such viruses in this group, one of which is CMV. Most people have been exposed to CMV sometime in their life, but typically, CMV does not cause symptoms of illness. However, in people with weakened immune systems, such as those living with HIV, CMV can cause illness and infection. Initially, CMV infection causes flu-like symptoms, fever, and fatigue. These symptoms usually resolve without intervention, and the person will feel better. CMV then lays dormant for years without causing symptoms or illness. Later, as the immune system weakens, CMV re-activates, causing new infections throughout the body.

- Symptoms—**CMV retinitis** (CMV that infects the retina of the eye) causes inflammation of the retina, resulting in visual changes, "floaters," diminished vision, blurred vision, and, in some cases, blindness. **CMV colitis** infects the gastrointestinal tract, resulting in *colitis* (inflammation of the bowels), *cholangitis* (inflammation of the bile duct), and ulcerations in the mouth, throat and/or rectum. CMV infections in the GI tract cause abdominal pain, fever, diarrhea, and weight loss.

- Risk Level — Most people have been exposed to CMV some time in their lifetime but will experience no ill affects from the virus. However, once the CD4 count falls below 50 cells/mm^3, the incidence of illnesses like CMV retinitis and CMV colitis increases dramatically.

- Prevention/Prophylaxis— Oral *gancyclovir* or *valgancyclovir* can be used as prophylaxis medications to prevent the first CMV infection in those patients at highest risk, specifically people with a CD4 count less than 50 cells/mm^3 or who have ever had a CD4 count less than 50 cells/mm^3.

- Treatment — The most effective treatment for both CMV retinitis and gastrointestinal CMV is the antiviral medication gancyclovir. Treatment is given intravenously in the acute stages of infection and then changed to the oral form of gancyclovir as a maintenance therapy to prevent reoccurrence of the infection. In some cases of CMV retinitis, antiviral medication implants are inserted in the affected eye directly at the site of infection in order to treat CMV retinitis locally.

Molluscum Contagiosum (molluscum)

Molluscum is caused by a very common virus that is a member of the group of viruses known as *Poxviridae*. Infection with this virus causes flesh-colored lesions seen initially in the genital area and thighs in people with normal immune systems. In people with weakened immune systems, the lesions can spread over the entire body, especially the face. Molluscum can be confused with genital warts, so definitive diagnosis is made by taking a small sample of the lesion and looking at it under the microscope (a biopsy).

- Symptoms— Molluscum causes small flesh-colored "bumps" or lesions first appearing in the inner thigh and genital area, spreading to the face and the rest of the body. These lesions are typically dome shaped with a hard white core in the middle. Some may have indentations in the middle. These lesions are most often painless but can itch intensely. Itching leads to scratching, increasing the risk of spreading the lesions to other parts of the body.

- Risk Level — Anyone exposed to molluscum, either by coming into contact with the skin of someone infected or by sexual contact with an infected person, can get this viral infection. In other words, people with any CD4 count can become infected. However, people with weakened immune systems are at higher risk of having disseminated (throughout the body) infection.

- Prevention/Prophylaxis — Using condoms during anal, oral, or vaginal sex is the best way to reduce the risk of molluscum infection. If you already have the infection, refraining from scratching the lesions will diminish the risk of spreading the molluscum all over your body. Using an electric razor has been known to diminish the incidence of molluscum spread by shaving with a blade.
- Treatment — Left untreated, molluscum will resolve over the course of several weeks to months, typically without leaving scars. If treatment is preferred, lesions can be frozen with liquid nitrogen one at a time. In many cases, molluscum infection will respond to HIV combination therapy.

Oral Hairy Leukoplakia (OHL)

OHL is caused by another virus from the herpesviridae family known as the Epstein Barr Virus (EBV). Found in the mouth, OHL is sometimes one of the first symptoms of HIV infection. The presence of OHL is an indication that the immune system has been damaged and is susceptible to other more serious infections.

- Symptoms — Leukoplakia is characterized by white patches on the sides of the tongue appearing similar to that of corrugated cardboard. Among the many folds are hair-like protrusions from which OHL got its name. Leukoplakia can be confused with thrush upon initial observation, the difference being that patches of leukoplakia can't be dislodged, as is the case with thrush. Usually diagnosis can be made simply by visual examination, but a biopsy can be done if necessary.
- Risk Level — As stated above, OHL can be one of the first symptoms of HIV infection. While it can occur at any CD4 count, people with CD4 counts less than 200 cells/mm^3 seem to have a higher incidence than those above 200 cells/mm^3.
- Prevention/Prophylaxis — Prophylaxis specifically for OHL is uncommon; however, patients taking fluconazole to prevent thrush have a lower incidence of OHL. Because HIV medications can help the CD4 count rise, people on HIV medication combinations have a lesser incidence of OHL as well.
- Treatment — OHL doesn't need to be treated unless it causes pain or interrupts eating, swallowing, or speaking. If treatment is indicated, the herpes medication acyclovir is used, in addition to HIV medication combinations.

Human Papillomavirus (HPV)

Papillomaviruses are a group of viruses that infect the skin and mucous membranes of humans and animals. There are over one hundred of such viruses called *Human Papillomaviruses (HPV)*. Some of these HPV are known to cause genital warts. While HPV is often thought of as one specific virus, there are actually several viruses that are considered HPV and cause genital warts. Other types of HPV can cause cervical cancer in women, anal cancer in men, and ordinary warts of the hands and feet. People living with HIV are most concerned about the HPV that causes genital warts, cervical cancer, or anal cancer. HPV is spread from person to person during unprotected sex. In most cases this very common virus is inactive, causing no symptoms of illness. However, for people with weakened immune systems, HPV can activate, causing genital warts, cervical cancers, and anal cancers.

- Symptoms—Once HPV activates it causes warts or "bumps" on the penis, vulva, in and around the anus, or in the mouth. If HPV infection results in cervical cancer or rectal cancer, symptoms of these conditions may include vaginal or rectal bleeding, vaginal or rectal discharge, and unusual appearing lesions. If symptoms of HPV infection occur they should never be ignored and should be addressed as soon as possible. Failure to do so could result in the progression of the HPV infection to the most serious forms of cancer.

- Risk Level—HPV can affect anyone, regardless of CD4 count. In fact, by the time we reach adulthood, most of us have been exposed and infected with HPV. People who engage in unprotected sex or have unprotected sex with multiple sex partners have a higher HPV incidence. Women infected with HIV are more at risk for HPV than women not infected with HIV. Cervical lesions as a result of an HPV infection seem to occur more frequently in women with CD4 counts less than 500 cells/mm^3.

- Prevention/Prophylaxis—Safer sex practices decrease the risk of spreading HPV from person to person. Regular physical exams can identify suspicious lesions early, meaning treatment of those lesions can begin earlier as well. In women, regularly scheduled PAP exams are done to identify abnormal cells. Typically, HIV-positive women, and those women with a history of previous abnormal PAP exams, should get PAPs every six months. HIV-negative women should get a PAP exam yearly. There is an HPV vaccine available to prevent HPV infection before it occurs. The hope is that by decreasing the incidence of HPV infection, the incidence of cervical cancer in women will decline as well.

- Treatment—Genital warts resulting from HPV can be treated in several ways. The warts can be frozen with liquid nitrogen and removed, or can be burned off with lasers. The topical prescription drug Aldara cream (imiquimod) can be applied directly to the warts if a less invasive method of treatment is desired. Any cancers that result from HPV require traditional cancer treatments, including radiation, chemotherapy, or surgery.

Herpes Simplex Virus (HSV)

HSV is a member of the herpesviridae family of viruses, along with varicella zoster virus (herpes zoster, VZV) and cytomegalovirus (CMV). Spread from person to person by way of sexual contact, the HSV, once infection has occurred, remains in the skin and nerve cells for life. Most often the virus is dormant and causes no symptoms. But in times of stress, when exposed to intense sunlight, or when suffering from a cold or other viral illness, the HSV can activate, causing painful, fluid-filled blisters. There are actually two types of HSV: HSV-1, which is the cause of oral herpes; and HSV-2, which is the cause of genital herpes. There is some evidence that HSV is a co-factor of HIV, meaning HSV may facilitate HIV infection of CD4 cells. There is also evidence that the presence of genital herpes increases the transmission risk of HIV.

- Symptoms— A herpes break-out may begin as a tingling, itching, or numb sensation of the skin or mucous membranes. This sensation is a result of the virus moving via nerve tracts, making their way to the skin. At the point of eruption, very painful, fluid-filled blisters form on the surface of the skin. These blisters eventually break open and crust over. The entire cycle from the initial sensation to out-break of the vesicles to complete healing can take up to two weeks.
- Risk Level— Herpes can strike anyone, regardless of the health of their immune system or whether or not they are HIV-infected. There is some evidence that suggests that herpes outbreaks are more frequent in people living with HIV.
- Prevention/Prophylaxis— In people who experience frequent herpes outbreaks, certain antiviral medications can be used to decrease the frequency of outbreaks. The medication *acyclovir* is one such antiviral that, if taken in low daily doses, can decrease the frequency of HSV outbreaks.
- Treatment — Oral antiviral medications such as *acyclovir*, *famciclovir*, and *valacyclovir* are used to treat acute herpes outbreaks. Keep in mind that these medications do not "cure" infections. Rather, they can shorten the time it takes for the outbreak to heal and reduce the severity of the outbreak. In the case of severe outbreaks or outbreaks involving the face or eyes, intravenous antiviral medications and hospitalization is required. There can be cases of herpes that are resistant to traditional medications. In those cases, stronger antiviral medications, such as *foscarnet*, are needed. Unfortunately, with stronger medication comes the risk of kidney and liver toxicity.

Herpes Zoster Virus (HZV)

Another member of the herpesviridae family, this virus is also known as the "chicken pox virus," "shingles," or "varicella zoster." Most people are infected with this virus as children in the form of chicken pox. After the initial infection, the zoster virus lies dormant in the body, reactivating later as itching, painful, fluid-filled blisters called shingles. Because the herpes virus resides along nerve tracts, shingles outbreaks are usually along the straight line paths of nerves. Because nerves are affected, the lesions itch and are usually very painful. In severe cases, hospitalization may be required. Varicella zoster is spread from person to person when someone with the virus coughs, sneezes, laughs or even talks in proximity to another person. Tiny water droplets containing virus are inhaled, spreading the infection from one person to another. In the case of shingles, transmission from person to person occurs by direct contact with the lesions.

- Symptoms— Very painful, itching, fluid-filled blisters appearing in linear patterns along nerve tracts of the flank, back, buttocks, and occasionally the face. Over the course of several days, the blisters break and crust over. Outbreaks of HZV can be precipitated by stress or irritation to the affected areas.

- Risk Level — Anyone can get HVZ, regardless of HIV infection or CD4 count. In order for someone to have a shingles outbreak, they have to have had chicken pox some time in their lifetime.

- Prevention/Prophylaxis— As is the case with herpes simplex, people who experience frequent HZV outbreaks use antiviral medications to decrease the frequency of outbreaks. The medication *acyclovir* can decrease the frequency and severity of HZV outbreaks if taken daily in low doses.

- Treatment — Oral antiviral medications such as *acyclovir*, *famciclovir*, and *valacyclovir* are used to treat outbreaks of herpes. Keep in mind that these medications do not "cure" infections. Rather, they shorten the duration of the outbreak while reducing the severity. In the case of severe outbreaks, especially those on the face and near the eyes, intravenous antiviral medications and hospitalization is required. There can be cases of herpes that are resistant to traditional medications. In those cases, stronger antiviral medications, such as *foscarnet*, are needed. But the stronger medication also has more risks, such as kidney and liver toxicity.

Progressive Multifocal Leukoencephalopathy (PML)

This viral infection of the brain is caused by the *JC virus* (JCV). The virus was first identified in 1971 and was named after the initials of a patient suffering from PML at the time the virus was isolated. Most people are exposed to JC virus at some point in their life. In the presence of a healthy immune system, the virus does no harm. However, in people with weakened immune systems, such as those living with HIV, JCV causes a potentially fatal infection of the brain known as *Progressive Multifocal Leukoencephalopathy*, or *PML* for short. PML most often appears after there has been significant damage to the immune system at the hands of HIV, occurring in people whose CD4 counts are less than 100 cells/mm^3. Before the advent of HIV medications, PML was fatal within a few months of contracting the infection. The Centers for Disease Control has classified PML as an *AIDS-defining illness*, meaning that if a person is diagnosed with PML, they are said to also have AIDS.

- Symptoms— Because PML affects the brain, symptoms reflect impairment of the central nervous system — loss of memory, seizure activity, visual disturbances, speech difficulties, and numbness or weakness of the arms, face and legs. Left untreated, these symptoms can progress to coma and eventually death.
- Risk Level — HIV-infected people with a CD4 count less than 100 cells/mm^3 are at the highest risk. In people without HIV, anyone with a significantly damaged immune system, such as cancer patients receiving chemotherapy, are at risk for PML.
- Prevention/Prophylaxis— While there is no specific medication that reduces the risk of PML, HIV medication regimens increase CD4 levels, which in turn strengthen the immune system, decreasing the risk of PML. Keeping the CD4 count higher than 100 cells/mm^3 is the best way to prevent PML.
- Treatment — As stated earlier, prior to the advent of HIV medications, PML killed its victims in just a few short months. Today, HIV medications that are able to cross the blood-brain barrier into brain tissue offer an effective treatment option for PML. HIV antiretroviral medications that cross the blood brain barrier include *lamivudine, retrovir (AZT), stavudine* and *nevirapine.*

The AIDS-Defining Illnesses

The previous sections described opportunistic infections commonly found in people living with HIV. Some of the most serious and life threatening opportunistic infections only occur after the immune system has suffered significant damage at the hands of HIV. The most serious of these illnesses are classified as *AIDS-defining* — meaning any HIV-positive person who has had one of these infections is henceforth classified as having AIDS.

At one point early in the epidemic, an AIDS diagnosis was a very significant milestone. There was no HIV test, so surveillance professionals used an AIDS diagnosis to monitor and track the epidemic. Tragically, an AIDS diagnosis also meant that the person was in the late stages of infection and had very little time to live. People diagnosed with AIDS would usually be very sick or near death. Those that weren't would quit their jobs, tie up loose ends in their life and wait for death. Simply put, an AIDS diagnosis was a death sentence.

Today, HIV testing allows for earlier diagnosis and more accurate surveillance. People are now being diagnosed before significant immune system damaged has occurred. The advent of HIV medications has lengthened the lifespan and slowed the progression of HIV to AIDS. In most people with an AIDS diagnosis, death is no longer imminent. In fact, people can live for years or even decades after an AIDS diagnosis, thanks to advances in HIV treatment and the treatment of opportunistic infections. In many cases, HIV medications can help the body rebuild the immune system — meaning that people at risk for AIDS-defining illnesses can actually rebound and be less at risk than they were when they were diagnosed as having AIDS.

In short, today an AIDS diagnosis is much less significant than it once was. It's merely a classification that helps surveillance agencies gauge how well we are doing in our fight to end the epidemic. Nevertheless, people living with HIV focus on AIDS as the benchmark in their own war on HIV. The media, the general public, and even some medical practitioners use the terms HIV and AIDS interchangeably. But, as we have discussed, they are not the same.

The following is a list of those illnesses classified as being AIDS-defining. Some we have covered already, others we will cover in future chapters.

- Candidiasis of bronchi, trachea, or lungs
- Cervical cancer (invasive)
- Coccidioidomycosis, Cryptococcosis, Cryptosporidiosis
- Cytomegalovirus disease (CMV)
- Encephalopathy (HIV-related)
- Herpes simplex (severe infection)
- Histoplasmosis
- Isosporiasis
- Kaposi's sarcoma (KS)
- Lymphoma characterized by swollen lymph nodes (lymphadenopathy)
- Mycobacterium avium complex
- Pneumocystis (carinii) jiroveci pneumonia (PCP)
- Pneumonia (recurrent)
- Progressive multifocal leukoencephalopathy (PML)
- Salmonella septicemia (recurrent)
- Toxoplasmosis of the brain
- Tuberculosis
- Wasting syndrome

In the coming chapter we will discuss other illnesses not caused by HIV directly, but which are illnesses that many people living with HIV have to battle as part of their life with the virus.

9

Associated Conditions

In the last chapter we discussed illnesses and infections that arise when the body's immune system has been damaged or weakened. We've discussed opportunistic infections that are a direct result of immune system damage at the hands of HIV. In addition to those infections and illnesses, there are other physical and mental health issues that commonly occur in people living with HIV. Some are a result of long-term use of HIV medications. Others are stress related, arising from the stress associated with an HIV diagnosis. And finally there are illnesses that, for one reason or another, are more common in people living with HIV. Let's explore some of the conditions that further complicate the life of a person living with HIV.

Lipodystrophy

As we have discussed in previous chapters, HIV-positive people are living longer due mainly to the introduction of HIV medications in the early 1990s. As we have also mentioned, many of the HIV medications have untoward effects on the body that emerge after long-term use. One of the most common problems associated with HIV medications is *lipodystrophy*. Lipodystrophy is a condition characterized by the redistribution of fat to the upper back ("buffalo hump"), the abdomen and the neck. Fat accumulations also appear as small fatty tumors (lipomas) throughout the body, and fat accumulation in the liver. As fat is distributed to areas around the body, it's lost in the extremities, face, and buttocks, leaving those areas looking very thin and malnourished.

Lipodystrophy was first identified in HIV-positive people around 1996. While aspects of the condition were identified earlier in the epidemic, true cases of lipodystrophy only emerged after 1996 when three-drug HIV medication regimens became common. It was at the Interscience Conference on Antimicrobial Agents and Chemotherapy (*ICAAC*), held in Toronto in 1997, when scientists first reported on patients who had developed increased fat deposits around their abdomen and the back of the neck; the problem of lipody-strophy had arrived in earnest.

Experts noticed that the first patients identified as having symptoms of lipodystrophy all had one thing in common: they had been treated with HIV medication regimens that included a drug from the class of HIV medications known as protease inhibitors (see chapter 7). As more cases emerged, the link between lipodystrophy and protease inhibitors strengthened. In fact, the connection was so strong that experts in the field of HIV care coined the term "*protease paunch,*" referring to the increased abdominal girth typically seen in patients diagnosed with lipodystrophy. However, eventually cases emerged in patients that weren't taking protease inhibitors. In fact, some patients being diagnosed with lipodystrophy had never taken protease inhibitors at all. Experts had to change their way of looking at lipodystrophy. Doing so has led to new theories to explain lipodystrophy.

One school of thought places the blame on hormonal changes common in HIV-positive people. HIV-positive people, especially men, often have abnormally low levels of the male hormone testosterone. While testosterone is a male hormone, both males and females produce the hormone naturally and need sufficient quantities in order to be healthy. One of the functions of testosterone is to generate and maintain lean muscle mass. With abnormally low quantities of testosterone, the body produces and stores fat instead of lean muscle. As a result, fat redistributes from the extremities, buttocks, and face to the abdomen, upper back, and along the jaw line — typical of the person diagnosed with lipodystrophy. Experts agree that this theory does explain the body's tendency to produce and store fat instead of lean muscle, a situation seen in the lipodystrophy patient. However, scientists point out that in some cases of lipodystrophy there is no evidence of abnormal hormone levels.

Another theory suggests that HIV medications interfere with fat metabolism. This theory does not single out the protease inhibitor class. Instead, this theory suggests that all HIV mediations interfere with fat metabolism to some degree. But again, this theory does not explain why some patients who have never been on HIV medications can show evidence of lipodystrophy.

Yet another theory suggests that HIV can contribute to insulin resistance, which in turn interferes with glucose metabolism. Glucose is the energy source of the cell. During glucose metabolism, sugars taken into the body are broken down so the cells can use them for energy. Insulin is a substance produced by the body that assists cells in their use of glucose as energy. If insulin resistance occurs, glucose is not used in the cells for energy. Instead, it is viewed as a surplus energy source and is stored in the form of fats throughout the body. In other words, when glucose metabolism is interrupted, serum (blood) glucose levels are abnormally high, meaning the body needs to store this excess energy and does so in the form of body fat.

Finally, there are some who believe lipodystrophy is just another complication of HIV. They explain that prior to HIV medications, HIV-positive people didn't live long enough for the signs of lipodystrophy to become evident. With the advent of HIV medications and longer life spans, the long-term effects of HIV infection begin to emerge — in this case, the signs and symptoms of lipodystrophy.

Typically, lipodystrophy in and of itself doesn't present an eminent danger to the HIV-positive person. However, there are some effects that result from the condition. For instance, most of us are aware of the fact that an excess of fat in the body can cause conditions that can be detrimental to health. Examples of these include high blood pressure, heart disease, diabetes, and elevated cholesterol and triglycerides in the blood. In addition to the metabolic problems just mentioned, there are physical problems with lipodystrophy, too. Many people who have lipodystrophy complain of neck pain, headaches, and, in extreme cases, difficulty breathing because of the fat build-up around their neck and upper back.

The concept of body-image is impacted, too. Lipodystrophy can have a negative impact on the emotional self, as well as the physical self. In other words, the physical changes that occur with lipodystrophy have emotional implications. The loss of fat in the face and extremities, and the subsequent redistribution of this fat to the neck and abdomen, result in the characteristic look of lipodystrophy. As does a person who loses a leg, the patient with lipodystrophy has an altered image of body and self. Many patients feel that the physical appearance of lipodystrophy makes them look "sick." Patients with lipodystrophy fear their appearance may spark health-related questions from friends, coworkers, or loved ones— questions they are not prepared to answer because of a fear their HIV diagnosis will become public. One of the greatest fears an HIV-positive person has is that his confidentiality will be compromised.

In addition to fear, some people with lipodystrophy feel their appearance is a constant reminder that they are sick with a chronic disease — a reminder that they are living with HIV. For many, living with their HIV diagnosis means struggling every day to go with a normal day-to-day life despite their HIV. Seeing their reflection in the mirror every day and their body changed by the effects of lipodystrophy becomes a constant reminder of their disease. Many choose not to think about their illness each day in an attempt to lead a "normal" life unencumbered by their illness. The characteristic look of lipodystrophy can, for some, make that very difficult. For others, this daily reminder is too much to bear, leading to emotional and mental health issues in addition to their lipodystrophy and HIV.

Fortunately, there is hope for those people affected by lipodystrophy. Unfortunately, there is no definitive cure for the condition. But there are a number of interventions that have proven to be effective in the treatment of lipodystrophy. One method of treatment is to use drug regimens that do not contain protease inhibitors. Many feel there is still a strong link between long-term protease inhibitor use and lipodystrophy. By changing medication combinations and thereby eliminating protease inhibitors from HIV regimens, one possible cause of lipodystrophy is removed. For some, this method is effective, while in others it doesn't seem to help at all. In fact, some people continue to have worsening lipodystrophy even without taking protease inhibitors. For some, eliminating protease inhibitors can slow lipodystrophy, only to have it return later even in the absence of protease inhibitors.

Another way to treat lipodystrophy is to stop HIV medications altogether. Obviously, this method is only an option for people with well-preserved immune systems. If this method is employed, frequent CD4 and viral load monitoring is absolutely essential to regularly assess the health of the immune system and the extent of HIV replication. Eventually, there is a good chance the HIV medications will need to be restarted in order to protect the immune system.

Some success has been seen in people using improved diet and regular exercise to treat lipodystrophy. By controlling the amount of fats in the diet — those fats in the form of triglycerides and cholesterol — the risk of developing lipodystrophy when compared to people with elevated body fat is much less. For those who can't lower their cholesterol and triglycerides by diet and exercise only, cholesterol-lowering medications can be prescribed. There is evidence that these drugs can lessen the extent of lipodystrophy in some people. Whether a diet low in cholesterol and triglycerides, and a lifestyle that includes regular exercise, effectively controls lipodystrophy or not, the benefits for the overall health of everyone, including HIV-positive people, are well documented. We will discuss this in detail in an upcoming chapter.

Some researchers believe that hormonal therapy, specifically testosterone, may be helpful in controlling the body changes of lipodystrophy. However, the value of hormonal therapy is not entirely clear. In addition, testosterone has its share of side effects that may negate any small improvement in lipodystrophy that may be gained from testosterone therapy.

While the aforementioned treatments or interventions to combat the causes of lipodystrophy can help to some degree, there are other options that address the physical changes of lipodystrophy. However, since these interventions do not address the underlying cause of lipodystrophy, the effects of many of these interventions are only temporary.

PLASTIC SURGERY

Tummy tucks, nose jobs, and breast enhancements are all the rage these days. Don't like your hips? Have them re-sculptured. Are your "love handles" getting out of hand? Just suck out a little of that extra fat. Skilled plastic surgeons can do wonders for our appearance and self-esteem. So it's not surprising that many HIV patients have turned to plastic surgeons to ease the symptoms of lipodystrophy. There are a few plastic surgery procedures that can help.

In the early 1980s a French plastic surgeon introduced a procedure using cannulas and high volume suction to evacuate large amounts of excess fat from the abdomen and thighs. The procedure, called liposuction, uses large amounts of fluid to break up fat deposits; and then that broken up fat is suctioned from the affected areas. In the case of lipodystrophy, liposuction has become a viable option. However, it's only effective for removing the fat that has been deposited at the back of the neck — often called a "buffalo hump." The reason being is that the "buffalo hump" is subcutaneous, meaning it is deposited directly below the skin. However, the fat deposits of abdominal lipodystrophy are in the abdominal cavity and are not subcutaneous. Therefore, liposuction is not an option.

So what is done with the excess fat that has been removed? In some cases, that fat can be transferred to the face to replace fat that has been lost around the cheeks. Simply put, the surgeon does a fat *transfer* from a place of excess fat to a place where fat has been lost. However, fat transfer is not without potential problems. There may not be enough fat to transfer to make a visible difference. In some cases there is plenty of fat to transfer but the results often appear unnatural or "lumpy." Finally, there is some evidence that the procedure itself stimulates more fat redistribution, meaning that, despite the fat transfer, redistribution will reoccur eventually and is often worse than before the procedure.

The last plastic surgery option is surgical implants. Similar to breast implants, these surgical implants can give shape and structure to the face, cheekbones, or buttocks misshapen by lipodystrophy. For instance, the sunken appearance of the cheeks after fat has been lost can be built up with surgical implants in order to reestablish the normal structure of the face. Surgical implants rebuild the areas and give structure where there was once only an absence of fat and a sunken appearance.

Like all surgical procedures, there are risks involved. Infection, anesthesia complications, bleeding, or procedural failures are all possibilities. In addition, because most insurance companies consider most plastic surgery procedures cosmetic, they are often not a covered service. And as we all know, surgery and the care required after the procedure can be very expensive. But despite all these potential problems, people with lipodystrophy have undergone the procedures discussed here, and for many the results have been positive.

Lactic Acidosis

The scenario has repeated itself hundreds of times since the advent of HIV medications. Aside from the typical nausea and occasional diarrhea HIV medication causes, the medication regimen is working well. Then, after taking the medications for a while, the HIV-positive patient begins to experience symptoms that include muscle pain, weakness, and worsening nausea and vomiting. Abdominal pain becomes a constant companion, as does pain, numbness, and tingling in the hands and feet. Finally, severe weakness sends the person to the emergency room, with subsequent admission to the hospital. This is the typical scenario of another HIV-related illness, *lactic acidosis.*

Our bodies are made up of trillions of cells, each one needing energy to carry on cellular functions. This energy is produced by the body during glucose (sugar) metabolism. This process occurs in the "power plant" of our cells called the *mitochondria*. In normal, healthy cells, the mitochondria produce the energy each cell needs every second of every day. The process of energy production also leaves behind a by-product known as lactic acid. Typically, the lactic acid is processed by the cell and eliminated as waste from the body. But in instances where the mitochondria have been damaged for some reason, lactic acid accumulates in our cells and our blood stream, resulting in the condition known as *lactic acidosis.*

But how do the cell mitochondria become damaged? In the case of people living with HIV, the exact mechanism of mitochondrial damage is not fully understood. There is one predominant theory that most HIV experts feel is the reason for HIV-related lactic acidosis. Beginning a couple years ago, experts started seeing lactic acidosis in association with the class of HIV medications known as Nucleoside Reverse Transcriptase Inhibitors (NRTIs) (see Chapter 7). In order to produce energy for the cell, the mitochondria need specific enzymes produced naturally in the body. NRTIs interfere with one of these enzymes, interrupting the mitochondria's ability to produce cellular energy and carry on cellular functions. One of these cellular functions removes lactic acid from the cell. If the cell loses that ability, lactic acid builds up to toxic levels within the cell, resulting in lactic acidosis.

The symptoms of lactic acidosis are mild at first. In fact, they can be so mild that some people assume they are coming down with a viral illness that will resolve after a couple of days. But left untreated, these mild symptoms will soon give way to the serious, life-threatening symptoms of lactic acidosis. A mild upset stomach gives way to severe nausea, followed soon after by frequent vomiting. A typical stomach ache becomes constant, severe abdominal pain. Fatigue and feeling "winded" becomes shortness of breath and difficulty breathing. Finally, a few minor aches and muscle stiffness become severe muscle pain and weakness. Because the symptoms of lactic acidosis can mimic or be very similar to other, less severe conditions, the most definitive way to diagnose lactic acidosis is by a blood test. The amount of lactic acid in a small sample of blood is measured in the lab. If the amount of lactic acid in the blood sample exceeds what's normally found in the blood stream, a diagnosis of lactic acidosis is made.

Experts agree. It's important to identify lactic acidosis as early in the course of the condition as possible. An early diagnosis and early intervention will lead to a more favorable prognosis. Anyone taking HIV medications should know their own body and be able to identify signs and symptoms that are out of the ordinary. Learn all you can about the medicines you take, and be alert for any signs or symptoms that may signal the onset of lactic acidosis. Once the problem develops, the only way to treat lactic acidosis is to stop NRTI therapy altogether. Some researchers are investigating enzyme replacement as a possible answer to lactic acidosis. More importantly, scientists are racing to develop new nucleoside analogue drugs that are less likely to cause mitochondrial damage, and new classes of drugs that attack HIV in an entirely new way. But for now, the key to being healthy is to recognize signs and symptoms of lactic acidosis and notify your doctor immediately if they do occur.

Peripheral Neuropathy

Some people describe peripheral neuropathy as a burning sensation in their hands and feet. Others say it's the sting of a thousand needles. It can be a searing pain or a cold, heavy numbness. Peripheral neuropathy can make each step a tenuous chore. While the experiences with peripheral neuropathy are all different, everyone who has ever suffered from the condition agrees: peripheral neuropathy is no fun.

Peripheral neuropathy (PN) is a condition of the peripheral nervous system. The peripheral nervous system is made up of the nerves outside of the spinal cord and brain. The peripheral nerves are primarily those that send impulses from the extremities to the brain. These are the nerves that are responsible for the sensations of touch, heat, cold and pain. Peripheral neuropathy results from damage to the insulating cover of the peripheral nerves. Think of your peripheral nerves as an electric wire composed of two parts — a copper wire covered with a plastic insulating cover. The electric current travels through the copper wire from one end of the circuit to the other. If anything comes in contact with the copper wire, the flow of electric current is interrupted. For that reason, the copper wire is insulated with a plastic cover. This plastic cover keeps the electric current flowing along the intended path. Peripheral nerves are much the same. The nerve impulses travel along the inner nerve fiber, and the outer covering of the nerve insulates the nerve, keeping the nerve impulse traveling along the intended path.

Damage to the protective covering of peripheral nerves can occur for many reasons. For instance, one of the long-term effects of diabetes is damage to the insulating cover of peripheral nerves. Poor nutrition and lacking certain vitamins can also cause peripheral neuropathy. In the case of HIV, peripheral neuropathy can result as one of the effects of HIV itself, or can occur as a result of long-term HIV medication use. Less common causes of peripheral neuropathy among HIV-positive people include viruses such as cytomegalovirus (CMV) or opportunistic infections such as Progressive Multifocal Leukoencephalopathy (PML).

Among the HIV population, the most common cause of peripheral neuropathy of those mentioned is the long-term use of HIV medications. The HIV medications most commonly associated with peripheral neuropathy are the nucleoside reverse transcriptase inhibitors (NRTIs) Hivid (zalcitabine), Videx and Videx EC (didanosine), and Zerit (stavudine). Other medications that cause neuropathy (but not as often) include the protease inhibitors Crixivan (indinavir) and Norvir (ritonavir). Not everyone taking these medications will suffer from peripheral neuropathy, but the possibility should be considered when putting together HIV drug combinations. Besides those HIV medications just mentioned, there are other medications commonly used in the care of HIV that may contribute to or cause peripheral neuropathy. They include *INH* (*isoniazid*), *Myambutol* (*ethambutol*), *Flagyl* (*metrodinazole*) and *Dapsone* (*diamino-diphenyl sulphone*).

Unfortunately, there is no cure for peripheral neuropathy. Even stopping the medications believed to be the cause of peripheral neuropathy may not relieve the symptoms or halt its progression. In some unfortunate cases, peripheral neuropathy becomes permanent even after removing the cause. However, there are ways to ease the symptoms, both medicinal and non-medicinal. The anti-convulsion drug *Neurontin* (*gabapentin*) is probably the most commonly prescribed drug to relieve the symptoms of peripheral neuropathy. The antidepressants *Elavil* (*amitryptyline*) and *Pamelor* (*nortriptyline*) increase peripheral nerve impulses, easing the numbness and tingling of neuropathy. Finally, in mild cases, non-steroidal anti-inflammatory medications such as *ibuprofen* (*Motrin, Advil*) can be used to relieve the pain of peripheral neuropathy. However, in moderate to severe cases, stronger pain relievers such as the narcotics *Vicodin* or *Fentanyl* are used. While these drugs are known to be addictive, studies have shown that the incidence of addiction and dependence are less in those people who truly need the narcotics for pain relief. Nonetheless, physicians prescribe these medications only after weighing the risks and benefits.

There are non-medicinal ways to ease the symptoms of neuropathy as well. Shoes should be loose fitting to maximize nerve impulses and blood flow to the extremities. Walking long distances or standing for long periods of time should be avoided. There have even been some documented benefits of wearing magnets in the shoes and socks of people with peripheral neuropathy. However, before investing any money on this method of symptom relief, great care should be used due to the high incidence of fraud associated with such non-conventional forms of treatment.

At the earliest sign of peripheral neuropathy symptoms, patients should consult with their doctor. Typically, the sooner the peripheral neuropathy is addressed the better chance the person has to recover from peripheral neuropathy. The longer the cause of neuropathy is left unaddressed, the more nerve damage will be done. In other words, if left untreated the chances are good that the peripheral neuropathy will become permanent. Eliminating the cause or causes before too much damage is done to the peripheral nerve sheaths is the key to recovery.

Depression

Everyone has had days during which they feel a little "blue." We have all been "down in the dumps" or felt "blah" at one time or another. But when these feelings become your daily companion, when there are more days of feeling "blue" then there are not, you may be suffering from a condition known as depression. And you would not be alone. In fact, depression affects more than 10 million Americans each year. One in four people will have an episode of depression some time in their lifetime. And if the physical stresses of HIV were not enough, depression is a very common condition among HIV population.

By definition, depression is an alteration in mood that affects a person's ability to function day to day. While short episodes of feeling down are considered normal variations in mood, longer-lasting feelings of despair are indicative of depression. Keep in mind the effects of depression are not only emotional. Physical manifestations, such as changes in appearance or behavior, are common. Physical illnesses such as indigestion, headaches, insomnia, and heartburn can all be part of depression as well. Depression is a serious illness with symptoms that should not be ignored. If ignored or left untreated depression can have catastrophic consequences.

While every cause of depression is not known, there are countless factors that can affect mood and emotional stability. Emotional stability is maintained by chemicals in the brain. If those chemicals go out of balance, alterations in mood will occur — specifically, depression. Chemical imbalances are triggered by life events such as losing a loved one, divorce, physical or emotional trauma, narcotic withdrawal, or chronic illness— HIV, for instance. Family history and genetics can also predispose a person to the chemical imbalances that cause depression. Finally, medications can cause the alterations in mood that result in depression, HIV medications included. The HIV medication known to increase the risk of depression is the medication Sustiva (efavirenz). In fact, many HIV specialists will also prescribe an antidepressant when prescribing an HIV regimen containing Sustiva.

As is the case with physical illnesses, there are early signs and symptoms that signal the onset of depression. Recognizing these early symptoms is the key to a favorable outcome. Diagnosing depression in its early stages means starting treatment earlier in the course of the disease. In most cases, early treatment translates to a less complicated course and a better prognosis. On the opposite end of the spectrum, untreated depression can progress to harmful and even life-threatening behaviors.

THE CORE SYMPTOMS OF DEPRESSION

There are a collection of symptoms that typically are at the root of most cases of depression. Subdued mood with a loss of energy or feelings of being "run down" are very common among those who are depressed. Often times, people with depression will lose interest in those activities they once found to be very enjoyable. People who are depressed find that concentration is difficult and that mental function is slowed. People will feel physically ill, with significant pain and muscle soreness. Finally, depressed people report decreased appetite and difficulty falling asleep and staying asleep.

Physical Symptoms

In addition to those symptoms considered core symptoms, there are other physical manifestations of depression, including headaches, excessive sleep, heartburn, stomach upset, indigestion, and unexplained weight loss. In addition, pain in the joints, muscles, or bones can be significant and debilitating, resulting in the inability or lack of desire to hold a job or attend school.

The Most Serious Symptoms

Depression can progress and have serious consequences if left untreated. Living day to day with such profound feelings of physical and emotional pain can become too much for a person to bear. Eventually, feelings of hopelessness give way to anxiety, guilt or helplessness. Feeling helpless and unable to shake the feelings of sadness, people search for a way to end their suffering. They try to find an escape from the pain. Unfortunately, many people choose the ultimate escape — they choose to end their life by suicide. Initially people will think about suicide as a way out but won't take the next step. However, if left untreated, the depressed person will eventually act on his feelings and attempt suicide. Unfortunately, in many cases, their attempts are successful.

But there is hope for those people suffering from depression. Treatment options are available that can help people dig themselves out from under the painful weight of depression. An assortment of antidepressants are available that have been found to be very effective. While many of the older antidepressants have significant side effects, the newer ones have fewer side effects that make taking them easier and, in turn, more effective. But medications alone aren't the answer. Antidepressants should be prescribed in conjunction with professional mental health counseling in order to find the root cause of the depression. Think of it this way. If you break your arm you take medication to relieve the pain. However, the medication does nothing to treat the root of the pain — the broken bone. For that, a cast is needed. So it is with depression. While antidepressants can relieve the unpleasant symptoms of depression, counseling will help you identify what has caused the symptoms of depression in the first place.

Elevated Cholesterol and Triglycerides

It's no secret; a well-balanced diet is one of the keys to a healthy life. One aspect of good nutrition is maintaining the right levels of fat in your blood. Two substances that we talk about when assessing the level of fat in your blood are cholesterol and triglycerides.

CHOLESTEROL

Cholesterol is a soft, fat-like substance that is produced in the liver. Cholesterol is a naturally occurring substance circulating in your blood stream and found in all of your body's cells. Cholesterol is also found outside of the body in foods such as meats, dairy products, and eggs. Cholesterol is needed for cell walls and membranes throughout the body, as well as for proper hormone, vitamin D, and bile (digests fat) production. But the body only needs a small amount of cholesterol — about what it makes naturally. Any additional cholesterol is deposited on the walls of blood vessels or accumulates in the liver. Think of the blood vessels as drain pipes in your kitchen sink and shower at home. When soap scum and food from your dishes builds up on the inside walls of those drains, the flow of water through the drain is slowed and will eventually stop altogether. The same is true when cholesterol clogs blood vessels. The flow of blood to vital organs such as the heart is slowed and eventually stopped as more and more cholesterol builds up on the vessel walls. As the flow of blood reaching your organs decreases, damage occurs. In the case of the heart, when the flow of blood to the heart muscle is stopped, the muscle is damaged and is no longer able to pump blood effectively; the person has had a *myocardial infarction*. In lay terms, the person has had a heart attack. And the reason is that there was too much cholesterol circulating in the blood. Simply put, cholesterol is a good thing to have — but only in the right amounts.

TRIGLYCERIDES

Triglycerides are the chemical form in which most fats exist, both in the foods we eat and in our body. They are often called "sugary fats" because they are composed of three fatty acids (fat molecules) and glycerol (a sugar molecule). Triglycerides in our blood are derived from fats eaten in foods or made in the body from other energy sources like sugars. Calories ingested in a meal and not used immediately by tissues for energy are converted to triglycerides and transported to fat cells to be stored. Hormones regulate the release of triglycerides from fat tissue so they meet the body's needs for energy between meals. Like cholesterol, the body needs triglycerides to function normally — but only in the right amounts. Excessive triglycerides in the blood stream increases the risk of serious health issues, particularly heart disease.

In many respects it's often not how much fat you have in your diet but what types of fat you are eating. For instance, eating the type of fat in red meat is much less healthy than eating the type of fat in fish. Eating the type of fat in a handful of macadamia nuts is much less healthy than eating the type of fat in a handful of unsalted almonds. Experts agree that too much fat is bad for your health, but there are types of fat that are actually better for you than others. In fact, some fats have been shown to decrease your risk of heart disease. It's important to know which are the "good fats" and which are the "bad fats." There are two types of cholesterol.

- High Density Lipids (HDL) — Also known as "good cholesterol," these lipids carry harmful fatty deposits away from cells and tissues to the liver for excretion from the body. An HDL that is too low actually increases your risk of heart disease.
- Low Density Lipids (LDL) — Also known as "bad cholesterol," these lipids account for most of the cholesterol in the blood. They carry cholesterol to the tissues by way of the blood vessels. Bad cholesterol is deposited on vessel walls, causing the vessels to become narrowed or clogged. Blood flow through narrowed or clogged vessels is diminished, making it more difficult to provide oxygen and nutrients to muscles, organs, and tissues throughout the body. Heart and vascular disease is a result of blood vessels clogged with bad cholesterol.

We have established that too much cholesterol and triglycerides circulating in the blood is bad for your health. There are many factors that can affect the levels of cholesterol in your blood. Some of these factors are out of our control. These factors include:

- a genetic tendency (a family history) to have high cholesterol levels;
- a genetic tendency to be more sensitive to lifestyle factors that can increase cholesterol;
- a family history of certain conditions or diseases (e.g., diabetes) that can increase cholesterol and triglycerides.

But many of the factors that can result in higher than normal cholesterol and triglycerides are under our control. They include:

- a diet high in fats and sugars (carbohydrates);
- little or no exercise;
- being overweight.

Many of the factors mentioned help to raise cholesterol and triglycerides in the HIV-positive person. Specifically, certain HIV medications interfere with the metabolism of fats, resulting in elevated triglycerides and cholesterol in the blood.

There is growing evidence that people taking protease inhibitors are at an increased risk of heart disease. Much of this increased risk is due to elevated cholesterol and triglycerides, caused by protease inhibitors. Specifically, cholesterol and triglycerides are elevated as a result of taking those protease inhibitors that are boosted with the medication Norvir (ritonavir). While most protease inhibitors can cause an elevation to some degree, it's boosted protease inhibitors that cause the most profound elevations. However, drug manufacturers are developing new protease inhibitors that do not affect triglycerides and cholesterol. One example of a newer protease inhibitor that does not elevate cholesterol or triglycerides is Reyataz (atazanavir). Even when boosted with Norvir (ritonavir), Reyataz (atazanavir) is less likely to elevate cholesterol and triglycerides when compared to other protease inhibitors that have been on the market longer.

There are steps you can take to keep your cholesterol and triglycerides under control. Treatment for elevated triglycerides and cholesterol usually starts with non-medicinal options—namely, diet and exercise. Typically, for people with elevated cholesterol and triglycerides, the instructions would be to reduce the amount of fats you eat. However, for people living with HIV, decreasing the amount of fats in your diet may not be so easy. Ironically, many protease inhibitors need the fats from food in order for the drug to be absorbed properly. Many HIV-positive people are underweight due to the effects of their disease. Limiting fat intake in these people may not be in their best interest. So in these special circumstances, making changes to the types of fat eaten is a better plan. An important way to do that is to learn how to read food labels. The Food and Drug Administration (FDA) requires food manufacturers to place labels on all their product packaging, itemizing what is contained in each product. The food labels list the ingredients of the product, how much fat, sugar, and protein is in the product, and how many calories are contained in each serving of the product. By reading and understanding labels, you can make sure you are eating the right types of fat in the proper amounts.

As we touched on earlier, some fats are better for you than others. For instance, animal fats, dairy fats, and foods containing palm oil contain cholesterol and triglycerides that are most detrimental to your health. Limiting these types of fats in your diet will help you cut down on the bad cholesterol and triglycerides in your body. On the other hand, certain fats, such as those contained in fish, flaxseed, and linseeds, are good for your overall health and should be eaten several times each week. Finally, replacing red meats with chicken, turkey, or tofu can cut down the amounts of bad fat that ultimately elevate your cholesterol and triglycerides.

As hard as we try, eventually it may take more than just changes in your diet to get your cholesterol and triglycerides under control. When dietary changes no longer maintain your cholesterol and triglycerides at an acceptable level, it may be necessary to consider cholesterol-lowering medications. There are several cholesterol-lowering drugs to choose from, depending on the needs of the patient and what types of cholesterol and triglycerides are too high. For example, one medication can lower your cholesterol, another lowers your triglycerides, and still others lower both. Some medications are designed specifically to lower bad cholesterol while elevating your good cholesterol.

In the case of the HIV patient, elevated cholesterol and triglycerides is most often a result of the medicines they are taking. Protease inhibitors such as Kaletra (lopinavir + ritonavir) and Lexiva (fosamprenavir), and non-protease drugs such as Sustiva (evaferenz) and Fuzeon (enfuvirtide), have been shown to elevate cholesterol and triglycerides, sometimes dramatically. Some of the newer protease inhibitors, namely Reyataz (atazanavir), do not affect cholesterol and triglycerides. In fact, scientists have placed a priority on developing HIV medications that have minimal impact on cholesterol and triglycerides. HIV specialists can choose to use HIV medications known to elevated lipids in the blood, or they can avoid those drugs and choose regimens that do not affect lipids at all. If the physician has no choice but to use one or more of those HIV medications that raise cholesterol and triglycerides, the physician will monitor those levels closely and will intervene with diet counseling or cholesterol-lowering drugs if necessary.

Avascular Necrosis (AVN)

The advent of HIV medications has lengthened the life span of HIV-infected people dramatically. Obviously that has always been the goal, leading to thousands of hours of research with the goal of finding a treatment for HIV. However, one unexpected result of longer life expectancy is the emergence of conditions, diseases, and illnesses that appear later on in the course of HIV. Before medicines, life expectancy of the HIV-positive person was not long enough for these conditions to emerge. One of those conditions that have emerged only since the age of HIV medications and longer life spans is *avascular necrosis (AVN)*. However, the risk of avascular necrosis is not simply a matter of a longer life. In fact, studies have shown that other conditions associated with HIV increase the risk of avascular necrosis. They include:

- long-term use of HIV medications;
- the use of steroids;
- a CD4 count less than 200 cells/mm^3 of blood;

- metabolic complications associated with HIV;
- living long-term with HIV.

So we know AVN is associated with long-term HIV diagnosis. Now let's take a look at what AVN is and what can be done about it.

Organs of the human body need to be well-nourished with the oxygen delivered to them by the blood. The same holds true for skin, hair, muscle and even bone. When that blood flow is disrupted, the body's systems are deprived of the oxygen and nutrients that are essential to their health and well-being. Such is the case in avascular necrosis. AVN is the death of bone cells due to an interruption of the blood supply. Without blood to nourish the cells, cellular death occurs. As more cell death occurs, the structure of bones, particularly the hip bone, weakens and will eventually collapse, causing pain and destruction of the bone, and with it a loss of hip function. As stated, AVN typically involves the hip bone and joint but can involve most any long bone, including the femur (leg), the humerus (arm) and the jaw.

There are many reasons blood flow to the hip is disrupted. For instance, trauma to the blood vessels that supply the hip will disrupt blood flow. Vascular disease narrows blood vessels of the hip, diminishing blood flow, which will eventually result in bone death. Finally, there is documented evidence that long-term exposure to certain medications, including protease inhibitors and steroids, can damage the blood vessels that supply the hip, once again resulting in cellular death and destruction of the hip bone and joint.

Typically, AVN starts with few or no symptoms. When symptoms do emerge, they are usually mild and vague, most often characterized by pain in the hip or groin. Unfortunately, because the initial symptoms are so mild, AVN can go undiagnosed for years. But eventually bone death and hip damage will become severe, causing significant pain that makes walking or bearing weight impossible. Fractures are common because the bone becomes brittle and weak due to bone death. In its most advanced stages, the hip can become so damaged that it resembles sawdust.

Because symptoms appear relatively late in the condition, they are not a suitable method of diagnosing AVN. Neither are basic hip x-rays. The most definitive way to diagnose AVN is by *Magnetic Resonance Imaging* (or *MRI* for short). MRI is a specialized type of imaging that uses magnetic and radio waves instead of x-rays to examine internal structures of the body. These waves are linked to a computer which creates very detailed images of body structures — in the case of AVN, the hip bone and joint.

Unfortunately, even after diagnosis there are few treatment options for those people found to suffer from AVN. Prescription narcotics are often needed for pain control, especially in advanced stages of the disease. There are medications that can reduce the swelling of surrounding tissues in an effort to decrease pain and eliminate the need for narcotics. Most often this intervention is only effective for the treatment of mild to moderate disease.

While there are a few options to treat the symptoms caused by AVN, there are very few options to actually treat the cause of AVN. And, unfortunately, once bone cell death occurs, that bone tissue is lost permanently. Remember, even if there was a way to grow bone to replace that which has died, the same diminished blood flow that caused the death in the first place persists. In order to halt the process of bone cell death, blood flow to the area must be improved. The way to do that is with vascular surgery. Blood flow to the area can be improved by using certain vascular surgery procedures. Some people will benefit from these vascular repairs, slowing or stopping bone cell death. However, while these procedures can be helpful in some people, the most effective way to manage AVN is through surgical hip replacement. Bones that make up the hip joint are replaced with prosthetic implants—in essence, rebuilding the entire hip joint. While there is some rehabilitation necessary after such surgery, hip replacement is the most effective way to treat AVN.

Hepatitis

Outside of the brain and heart, the liver is the most vital organ in the human body. When liver disease strikes it can be catastrophic for the individual. The liver can fall victim to many types of illnesses, infections, and diseases. One such condition that is common among those people living with HIV is *hepatitis*. To understand exactly what hepatitis is, let's break down the word. The *Online Etymology Dictionary* defines the word hepatitis as follows: "*Hepatitis — from the Greek 'hepatos' meaning liver and 'itis' meaning inflammation.*"

So, as the origin of the word indicates, hepatitis is an inflammation of the liver. The reasons for the inflammation are many. For instance, exposure to chemicals or toxic substances can damage liver tissue, causing inflammation. Excessive use of alcohol, or diseases of the gall bladder or pancreas, can also cause the inflammation of hepatitis. The metabolism or breakdown of certain medications by the liver, including some HIV medications, can place stress on the liver, once again causing inflammation. Finally, one of the most common causes of hepatitis, and one that can potentially be fatal, is viral infection. In other words, viral infections cause tissue damage, inflammation, and liver dysfunction. Let's explore the types of hepatitis that most commonly affect HIV-positive people.

VIRAL HEPATITIS

There are several types of viral hepatitis, some more common than others. Some are specific to certain geographic areas, and others are found all over the world. Some have vaccines to prevent their spread, and others do not. Let's take a look at the three most common forms of viral hepatitis: hepatitis A, B, and C.

Hepatitis A

This type of hepatitis can affect anyone. There can be isolated cases, but usually cases of hepatitis A appear in clusters. In some parts of the world, hepatitis A epidemics are widespread, involving large numbers of people. Hepatitis A is primarily a disease related to personal hygiene and sanitation conditions. This type of hepatitis is caused by the hepatitis A virus found in the feces of people infected with hepatitis A. It's spread from person to person by coming in contact with the stool infected with hepatitis A. Most people come in contact with hepatitis A by ingesting contaminated food — contaminated by poor hand washing, hygiene, or sanitation when preparing the food. Typically, the food was contaminated with hepatitis A because an infected person did not wash their hands after using the bathroom. Their contaminated hands come in contact with the food being served to others. Less common in the general public but common among some population groups is hepatitis A exposure during oral and anal sex. For instance, men who have sex with men have a greater risk of hepatitis A because they engage in anal sex routinely.

Thankfully, hepatitis A can be prevented and the risk reduced by doing a couple things. Good hand washing before and after using the bathroom, and before handling and preparing food, can reduce the spread of hepatitis A significantly. Another means of reducing the risk of hepatitis A infection is the hepatitis A vaccine. This series of two injections over the course of six months to one year has proven to be very effective in stimulating an antibody response that confers immunity to hepatitis A. This vaccine is particularly important to men who have sex with men, whether they are HIV positive or negative, because of their risk of hepatitis A from anal sex.

The symptoms of hepatitis A are similar to symptoms of many liver diseases. The symptoms are those of liver dysfunction and liver failure. These systems include:

- jaundice (yellowing of the skin and whites of the eyes);
- fatigue;
- abdominal pain;
- loss of appetite;
- diarrhea;
- nausea;
- fever.

The treatment of these symptoms depends a great deal on their severity. Most often, treating the symptoms and employing comfort measures is the extent of treatment. Meanwhile, the hepatitis A infection itself is allowed to run its course without treatment.

Hepatitis B

The virus that causes hepatitis B can produce life-long disease, resulting in scarring (cirrhosis), liver tissue damage, or even death. The mode of transmission differs from that of hepatitis A. Hepatitis B is spread from person to person by exposure to infected bodily fluids during sexual intercourse, needle sharing, needle sticks, and during delivery by a pregnant woman positive for hepatitis B. While hepatitis B can strike anyone, there are groups of people that are at a higher risk of infection than others. These groups include:

- people who have unprotected anal, oral, or vaginal sex;
- people who inject drugs and share needles and syringes;
- newborn children of infected mothers;
- and healthcare workers that are potentially exposed to infected bodily fluids or infected needles and syringes.

About 30 percent of all people infected with hepatitis B have no symptoms at all. If symptoms are present they include:

- jaundice (yellowing of the skin and eyes);
- abdominal pain;
- nausea and vomiting;
- dark urine;
- fever.

As you recall, hepatitis A is usually left to run its course untreated. The same can't be said for hepatitis B. There are medications available to treat hepatitis B. In fact, some of the medications used are the same medicines used to treat HIV, only in smaller doses. For instance, Epivir (lamivudine) is prescribed at 100mg daily to treat hepatitis B, but 300mg daily to treat HIV. There are medications that have been developed specifically for the treatment of hepatitis B. One such drug is called Baraclude (entecavir). In addition to treatments, there is a preventative vaccine. In fact, the hepatitis B vaccine is now part of the standard vaccination schedule for young children. Unfortunately, because some HIV-positive people have significantly weakened immune systems, the hepatitis B vaccine does not always confer immunity. In other words, because the immune system is so weak, the hepatitis B vaccine fails to cause the immune response necessary to confer immunity.

Hepatitis C

Approximately 170 million people worldwide are thought to be infected with the hepatitis C virus. Four million of those are from the United States. Sadly, a majority of people living with hepatitis C have no idea they are infected. In fact, so many people are infected but unaware that some experts refer to hepatitis C as the "silent epidemic." The phrase was coined to describe the asymptomatic nature of hepatitis C. The infection can persist for years without any symptoms at all. In fact, 80 percent of all people with hepatitis C are symptom free. If and when symptoms do occur they are similar to those seen in hepatitis A and B: jaundice, abdominal pain, fever, nausea, fatigue, dark urine, and loss of appetite.

Hepatitis C is spread from person to person by exposure to hepatitis C–infected blood. This typically occurs when sharing needles to inject recreational drugs; when receiving blood products prior to 1992 or clotting factors prior to 1987; by needle stick injury for those in the healthcare setting; or during childbirth involving a hepatitis C–infected mother. The fact that most people infected with hepatitis C experience no symptoms should not lead anyone to believe the infection is minor. In fact, hepatitis C causes chronic liver disease in about 70 percent of infected people, and will be fatal in many of those cases. Furthermore, hepatitis C is the leading indicator for liver transplant.

Unfortunately, there is no vaccine to immunize against hepatitis C, as there is for hepatitis A and B. Instead, people need to take precautions to prevent infection. These precautions include:

- not sharing needles or drug paraphernalia with others;
- not sharing any personal items that could be contaminated with blood (e.g. razors and toothbrushes);
- those who choose to get a tattoo or body piercing should make certain it's done by a professional tattoo artist using accepted health practices and proper sanitary techniques;
- a condom should be used with each oral, anal, or vaginal sexual encounter, regardless of how slight the risk is.

There are medications to treat hepatitis C, but adhering to a hepatitis C drug regimen requires a great deal of commitment. Side effects are common, can be very unpleasant, and in many people the benefit of the treatment is not entirely clear. When deciding if hepatitis C medications are indicated, doctors weigh the potential benefits of treatment versus the potential side effects. The current treatment of choice is a combination of two medications, pegylated interferon and ribavirin. This combination suppresses the virus in 50 to 80 percent of the people for whom it's prescribed.

Drug-Induced Hepatitis

In addition to viral hepatitis, which we have just discussed, there are also non-viral causes of hepatitis that affect the HIV-positive population. The most common non-viral hepatitis is drug-induced hepatitis. In addition to HIV medications, there are over 1000 other hepatotoxic (liver toxic) drugs on the market that can also cause hepatitis. These medications are typically broken down and metabolized by the liver. This process can place significant stress on the liver, causing inflammation and, in some cases, liver tissue injury. Medication-induced hepatitis can be very serious, and in some cases can cause complete liver failure.

Typically, drug-induced hepatitis will resolve after the drug or drugs causing the problem are discontinued, most often without permanent liver injury. However, in some cases the damage to the liver does not resolve even after stopping the medications. In the most severe cases of drug-induced hepatitis, liver injury can be so significant that liver failure can occur, requiring a liver transplant to save the life of the individual.

There are three reasons why drugs cause hepatitis. First, there are certain drugs that by their nature can be toxic to the liver. Taken in the prescribed dosages, the medications are non-toxic and do no harm. However, if these drugs are taken in amounts that exceed recommended doses they can damage the liver. Typically, the liver will break down these drugs into non-toxic by-products. In the case of medications that are "liver toxic," liver damage occurs after the medications are taken, in higher-than-recommended doses. In this instance, instead of the liver breaking down the drug into non-toxic by-products, the opposite occurs. When excess medication is taken the liver breaks down the non-toxic drugs into toxic by-products, resulting in liver damage.

There are other drugs that trigger an unexpected hypersensitivity to the drug, which results in hepatitis. This type of hepatitis is not related to dose, meaning the hypersensitivity is unexpected and can occur at any dose. Typically, this type of hepatitis does not occur until the person has been taking the drug for a prolonged period of time. How long after beginning the medication depends on the specific drug and the person for whom it's prescribed.

Finally, drug-induced hepatitis can be made worse or more likely to occur due to several external factors. These factors include age, genetics, certain illnesses and diseases (including HIV), smoking and the use of alcohol. Some of these factors can be controlled by the individual — smoking or drinking alcohol, for instance. Others, like genetics, age, and gender, are out of the control of the individual.

Wasting

Wasting syndrome has been a complication of HIV infection since the epidemic emerged in the 1980s. The thin, drawn appearance characteristic of wasting syndrome became the face of AIDS early on. In addition to being a complication of HIV infection, wasting can be a complication of many of the serious opportunistic infections that occur when the immune system is damaged by HIV. In fact, HIV wasting is considered an AIDS-defining illness by the Centers for Disease Control (CDC), meaning that if someone is diagnosed with HIV-related wasting they are considered to have AIDS.

Technically speaking, wasting is defined as a 10 percent loss of body weight, accompanied by diarrhea, fever, and often times a CD4 count less than 100 cells/mm^3 of blood. However, wasting can be seen in people with CD4 counts greater than 100 cells/mm^3 as well. Wasting is the result of one of three causes.

DISTURBANCES IN METABOLISM

Changes in the way the body metabolizes food results in the inadequate absorption of nutrients needed to maintain body weight. HIV can cause hormone deficiencies that can change the way food is metabolized. In wasting syndrome, muscle is burned for energy instead of fat due to hormonal changes that have interrupted normal metabolism. Cytokines are proteins that produce inflammation. People who are HIV positive have large amounts of cytokines, which makes the body more fats and sugars and less proteins. This lack of protein production contributes to wasting.

Hormone deficiencies can also affect metabolism. The deficiency of hormones, specifically the hormone testosterone, does contribute to wasting. While testosterone is a male hormone, both males and females normally have testosterone in their body. One role of testosterone in both men and women is to generate and maintain lean muscle mass. Inadequate levels of testosterone, combined with changing metabolic function, results in lean muscle mass being lost and not easily replaced. The result is a loss of lean muscle mass and continued wasting.

POOR NUTRITION

Many factors lead to a state of poor nutrition. Diminished appetite, coupled with increased caloric needs, leads to weight loss. In other words, even though the body needs more calories to fight HIV, a poor appetite makes it hard for the person in take in those calories. Nutrients are absorbed through the intestinal tract. Infections of the intestinal tract or other intestinal disorders can interfere with that absorption, further contributing to the wasting problem.

LOW FOOD INTAKE

Poor appetite is common among HIV-positive people. This, combined with the gastrointestinal side effects of some HIV medications, make it difficult for the HIV-positive person to take in the required calories each day. Plus, any disease state, including HIV, increases your caloric needs. Taking in those calories is made very difficult because of poor appetite. Finally, opportunistic infections, such as thrush and apthous ulcers inside the mouth, make eating difficult because of the pain they cause.

Wasting is not easily reversed. Treating the underlying opportunistic infections, gastrointestinal illnesses, and HIV itself will help slow and, in some cases, reverse wasting. Nutrition can be maintained with high-calorie nutritional supplements. Many HIV treatment programs utilize registered dieticians to assist their patients in the development and maintenance of a healthy diet. Testosterone can be replaced using hormone injections or transdermal patches. Anabolic steroids have been used as well to increase and maintain lean muscle mass. Finally, in those patients whose poor appetite prevents them from eating a healthy diet, appetite stimulants are used to allow patients to take in more calories. But simply increasing calories is not enough. The type of calories is important, too. For instance, increasing your caloric intake by eating 800 calories of ice cream is not nearly as helpful as eating 800 calories of protein in the form of fish.

As you can plainly see, people living with HIV and AIDS have to deal with many illnesses and infections, in addition to their HIV. In fact, so much progress has been made in the treatment of HIV that often times it's the other illnesses associated with HIV, such as hepatitis or wasting, that cause the most problems. As people continue to live longer, new and more challenging conditions that will challenge the HIV specialist and their patients are certain to emerge. It's the various associated illnesses that go along with HIV that cause experts to agree that the best way to treat HIV and AIDS is to treat the entire person — physical, mental, and emotional.

Our next chapter discusses the whole body concept of treating HIV and AIDS. Since the emergence of the disease, experts have learned that the best HIV treatment programs are the ones that follow this concept when caring for their patients. Let's see what that entails.

10

Treating the Whole Person

HIV affects all aspects of a person's life — physical, psychological, social and spiritual. For that reason, HIV care should address all those areas as well. So often care is centered on the physical aspects of HIV, leaving other dimensions of the individual unattended. Without addressing all the effects of HIV, both physical and emotional, people have significant difficulty living with the disease. Since the early years of the epidemic, experts agree that HIV-positive people need care that encompasses all aspects of a person — physical, emotional, and spiritual.

Professional counseling, as a member of a group or as an individual, can provide support and teach coping methods that will help a person deal with the day to day stress of HIV. Less structured methods of social support — those in the form of friends and family — help the HIV-positive person cope with the various issues associated with each stage of the disease. Psychosocial support in any one of these forms decreases the incidence of mental illness such as depression, and helps people cope with their new diagnosis and the adjustment period that follows. Continued support throughout the course of the disease will assist the HIV-positive person to live with a chronic disease, to persevere as the disease progresses, and finally to handle end-of-life issues prior to death. Ultimately, the person who needed the support of others becomes the support for others

As we know, an HIV diagnosis brings prejudice, stigma, fear, isolation and guilt. Psychosocial support helps the individual cope more effectively with these issues and assists in decision making surrounding HIV care. Without psychosocial support, prejudice, fear and other negative feelings will overwhelm even the strongest person, making a life with HIV even more difficult.

In addition to the obvious physical manifestations of HIV and the psychosocial issues we just discussed, HIV creates economic issues as well. Chronic illness often results in lost work, lost wages, and ever-increasing healthcare costs. Lack of employment also means medical and prescription coverage may be gone or inadequate. Finally, without adequate income, permanent housing is jeopardized, which in turn can impact medication adherence, nutrition, and overall health. But issues like these are not limited to those people with poorly-controlled HIV or people who are sick. Even if your health is good enough to maintain employment, the prejudice, fear, and ignorance of employers may prevent securing employment at all.

Personal relationships are not immune to the effects of HIV. Disclosing your diagnosis to a loved one is probably the most difficult thing you will ever have to do. A loving, supportive response to HIV disclosure is not guaranteed. In fact, HIV infection can and does tear relationships apart for a myriad of reasons. For example, if a man is married and is diagnosed with HIV, the wife is sure to ask where that infection came from. Did the man have a sexual encounter outside of the marriage? Does the man have a drug problem that his wife didn't know about? What about the gay man who has done well to hide his homosexuality from his family? Disclosing his HIV diagnosis may jeopardize his secret. His family will not only have to deal with his HIV diagnosis but also deal with the realization that their son or brother is gay. Simply put, disclosing an HIV diagnosis may necessitate revealing secrets as well, secrets that can stress or destroy a relationship.

Chronic illnesses such as HIV can impact relationships in other ways as well. Just like the newly-diagnosed person experiences fear, confusion, and denial, so will loved ones close to that person. These feelings can stress a relationship a great deal. It's for all these reasons that HIV care that addresses the whole person is absolutely essential. Let's look a little closer at the psychosocial aspects of HIV.

Grieving After Diagnosis

Grieving is a process that most people will experience at least once in their life. When we think of grieving, most of us think about the death of a loved one or maybe a divorce from a spouse. However, grieving is an emotion that most people experience when they get their HIV diagnosis for the first time. Like the death of a loved one, an HIV diagnosis signals a loss—the loss of your good health, a loss of control over your future, and a loss of the life you once had. Grieving is a process we all go through to cope with a loss in our life, be it the loss of a loved one or the loss of our health.

Dr. Elizabeth Kübler-Ross did a great deal of work in the field of grief and how people deal with loss. Her stages of grief have been the standard for understanding the grieving process since 1969 when she published her work *On Death and Dying*. The work deals with grieving and the stages we go through in times of a loss. Remember, the person with the new HIV diagnosis is not the only person who will experience grief. Loved ones, family, and friends will also go through these stages of grief as well. Learning to recognize these stages in yourself and loved ones will help all of you grieve more effectively. Let's look at Kübler-Ross's stages of grief to see how they apply to a new HIV diagnosis.

SHOCK

The initial reaction to hearing bad news, such as being diagnosed with HIV, is shock. Initially, there may be no reaction to the bad news at all. It's common for people to sit and stare, detaching themselves from the situation at hand. Others may just nod and appear accepting of the news. Still others may act as if the news of their diagnosis is no big deal. Internally, the person has mentally blocked out the news in an effort to protect themselves from something they do not wish to hear. Shock can impede understanding and retention of the news delivered. Often the diagnosis has to be repeated several times before the person is actually fully aware of what is being said and the gravity of the news being delivered. Physically, this stage of grief can be accompanied by tremors, nausea, vomiting, or sweating. Have you ever heard the term "you look like you've seen a ghost"? This phrase refers to the pale appearance common to someone in the first stage of grief. To ease the impact and duration of the shock stage of grief, HIV disclosure should be done in a private setting, allowing for the free expression of feelings that surface after hearing the news of their diagnosis.

DENIAL

After the initial shock of learning your diagnosis, the stage of denial begins. During this stage the validity of the HIV diagnosis is questioned. Simply put, the person receiving their diagnosis refuses to believe that what they're being told is true. Since they don't believe the diagnosis they carry on with their life as if nothing has happened. Unfortunately, this can be a dangerous thing to do. We know from earlier chapters that getting into care is the key to a healthy prognosis. By denying your diagnosis you delay healthcare, which will ultimately affect your prognosis in a negative way. So strong is the power of denial that many times physical symptoms miraculously disappear or resolve by themselves. It's not uncommon for the diagnosed and their loved ones to question the validity of the test results. Because they doubt the diagnosis, loved ones offer little support at this time. In fact, their denial may even reinforce feelings of denial the diagnosed person may be having.

ANGER

This stage is a direct result of repressing emotions that have developed during the first two stages of grief. This stage is characterized by an outpouring of emotion and grief in the form of verbal outbursts and other expressions of anger. It's during this stage that the diagnosed asks, "Why Me?" Their anger is usually directed toward a person nearby or to a person not infected or affected by HIV. The question "Why not you?" repeats itself over and over in the mind of those who grieve. Upon learning their loved one has been diagnosed with

HIV, people get angry and many times direct that anger at the HIV-positive person. If you have disclosed your status and the people you just told appear angry or direct anger toward you, try not to take this personally. This is a normal expression of grief by a person thinking they have lost someone very near and dear to them. As much as it feels like a personal attack, it is simply a normal expression of grief.

BARGAINING

After the anger has subsided and the pent up emotion has been released, bargaining begins. It's at this stage in the grief cycle that the person grieving tries to make a deal with a higher power. For instance, the person grieving will think something to the effect of "I'll clean up my life if you make this all go away," or "I'll eat right and exercise if you just let me be healthy." Bargaining, for the most part, is not an overt process where the grieving person stands in front of their doctor trying to make a deal. Instead, bargaining takes place in the mind of the one grieving, making private pacts with his or her god. It's quite common for the newly-diagnosed person to feel guilt or a sense of being punished for something they feel they've done wrong — an extramarital affair, drug use, or a gay lifestyle. This sense of guilt feeds into the bargaining stage of grieving. If a person feels they are being punished, then refraining from that which they feel is wrong will set things straight in their mind. In other words, the person bargains by asking his or her god for good health if they refrain from the activity they feel is wrong or immoral. Unfortunately, the guilt that emerges in this stage is often long-lasting and can impede a person's progress toward accepting their disease and moving on with their life.

In some cases, bargaining can take on another, less obvious face. Bargaining can also be in the form of seeking alternative therapies or experimental medications that may cure. In other words, the person bargains by showing they will do anything to stay healthy. For most, bargaining is a request for a second chance. In actuality, it is a form of hope that the bad news, in our case the HIV diagnosis, is reversible and will just go away if we do the right things with our life.

DEPRESSION

While bargaining is a product of denial, depression signals that the grieving person is moving toward acceptance. The inevitability of their new diagnosis "sinks in," and reluctantly the person accepts what has happened and what is going to happen. While anger and bargaining are very animated and outgoing, depression is isolated and lonesome. They turn away from support, treatment, or any outside help being offered to them. In this stage, people see very little hope for their future, seeing only illness, suffering, and despair before them. This stage can be a dangerous one. The depression in this stage can be so profound that people seek an escape from their diagnosis and their suffering. Some choose substances such as alcohol or drugs. Others will seek the ultimate escape — suicide. People in this stage are vulnerable to such extreme actions because of feelings of hopelessness, isolation, and withdrawal. For this reason it's important for loved ones to continue offering support even when those grieving refuse that support. Without support, the person is sure to slide further into a depression from which escape will be very difficult.

TESTING

It's during this stage that the grieving person begins to realize that he or she can't stay depressed forever. There comes a realization that surviving their new diagnosis will only be possible if there is acceptance. The person searches for actions that can be taken in an effort to cope with their new diagnosis. For instance, during this stage the newly-diagnosed begins their HIV care as a first step in dealing with their diagnosis. In most cases this stage can progress only with the support of loved ones and professionals. As the grieving person takes steps that prove beneficial and successful, he or she realizes that the steps being taken are better than the depression that they had been experiencing. Each successful step toward acceptance breeds another step.

ACCEPTANCE

This final stage of grieving is one of stability. The grieving person has advanced to a point where he or she is ready to move on with their lives. In the case of the newly-diagnosed, they will continue their HIV care and strive to incorporate their illness into their lives. As their grief process stabilizes, they will be ready to offer support to others. In some instances the newly-diagnosed are the support for the people to whom they disclosed their illness. Now having passed through all the stages of grieving, the loved one can be a support person for the person who is newly-diagnosed.

Keep in mind that people who are grieving can move in and out of stages more than once. Many times people will experience the stages of grief out of order or will experience more than one stage at a time. People can get stuck in one stage or skip a stage altogether. There is really no right or wrong way to grieve. While there are stages we all go through, how we pass though those stages is unique for each of us. The most important thing to keep in mind is that newly-diagnosed people and their loved ones will experience grieving of some sort. Coping with that grief will take time and support from those around them and one another.

Fear and Anxiety

Fear and anxiety are two common emotions experienced by the HIV-positive person. Especially in those early days immediately following diagnosis, fear and anxiety can be overwhelming for many people. The root of fear and anxiety in the HIV-positive person stems from the unknown. How will HIV change my life? How long will I live? Will I be sick all the time? All these questions are common for the newly-diagnosed person. Not knowing the answer to these questions causes anxiety. Assuming the worst creates fear. Not knowing what to expect after an HIV diagnosis, and fearing what others may think of you after having been diagnosed, only adds to the fear and anxiety.

While fear and anxiety are emotional conditions, they also cause physical symptoms. An elevated heart rate; rapid, shallow breathing; nausea; and interrupted sleep patterns can all occur in the midst of fear and anxiety. Additionally, a person suffering from fear and anxiety can experience profuse sweating, agitation, nervousness, shortness of breath, and dizziness. There are ways, however, to control or limit feelings of fear and anxiety. They include:

- Learn as much about HIV and AIDS as possible. Understanding the disease will ease the fear and anxiety by shedding some light on the unknown. Understanding the biology of HIV and its typical course will give some hint as to what the future with HIV holds. Fear is a product of the unknown. Decreasing the unknown will also decrease your fear.
- You will have questions about your disease. Make sure you get them answered to your satisfaction by your HIV specialist at your next visit. When questions arise, write them down. Take the list of questions to your next visit with your HIV specialist. The old adage "knowledge is power" is absolutely right. By better understanding your illness you are better able to control your fear and anxiety.
- Seek out emotional support in the form of friends, family, or loved ones. Find HIV-related support groups in your community. It's always helpful to speak with people experiencing feelings and emotions similar to your own. Learn from their experiences, and they can learn from yours.
- Once you have learned to control your fear and anxiety, reach out to someone else and offer to help. Volunteer at an HIV agency or in the HIV care program managing your disease. Helping others and being active in the HIV community empowers you, which in turn helps manage your fear and anxiety.
- If fear and anxiety persist after trying the above interventions, it may be time for a medicinal option. Anti-anxiety medications such as Ativan (lorazepam) or Valium (diazepam) can help, but have many side effects and the potential for dependence. Because of potential problems, drugs like

Ativan and Valium are intended for short-term use only. Your HIV specialist should consider these risks before prescribing anti-anxiety drugs. If an anti-anxiety medication will be needed long-term, you should consider professional counseling in addition to the medications. Taking medications such as Valium or Ativan is like putting a band aid on a cut. It will cover the wound but will do nothing for healing. Professional counseling can identify the causes of the fear and anxiety and treat that cause. If needed, there are medications that treat the cause rather than just masking the symptoms (as does Ativan and Valium).

Stress

We all experience stress in our everyday lives: the stress of a traffic jam; the stress of debts that need to be paid on time; the stress of raising three teenage daughters. Stress can be uncomfortable and unpleasant, but in many ways stress pushes us to succeed and helps us get things done. Stress can be an incentive to push forward, but only if we are able to control the amount of stress and how we react to it.

The causes of stress are unique to each one of us. We need to recognize what causes our stress and learn to cope before it gets the best of us. As you learn to recognize your stressors you will develop coping mechanisms that help manage stress. Learning what causes stress in your life allows you to take measures to minimize those causes and, in turn, decrease your stress. Here are just a few ideas how you can manage your stress.

- Physical activities, such as exercise, walking, or swimming, can help relieve the anxiety, nervousness, and anger characteristic of stress. Physical activity can help relieve tension created by stress, and it's an excellent way to improve your health as well.
- Take care of your body. Eat a healthy diet; get plenty of exercise and enough sleep. If you are irritable because you lack sleep, then you will be ill equipped to deal with the stress of your disease. If stress is interrupting your sleep patterns, talk to your doctor. He or she can suggest ways to improve your sleep and, if needed, can prescribe medications that will help you get the sleep you need.
- Develop a support system of people you trust and who care about you. Talk to them about your stress. Talking about your stress with others is therapeutic, and the people in your support system may suggest ways to deal with stress that you have not tried or considered.
- A good cry can be very helpful. It's a means of releasing the tension that builds during periods of stress. Relieving tension is the key to relieving stress. Tension prevents the body and mind from relaxing. Relaxation

allows us to recharge our batteries, so to speak, and in doing so it allows us to more effectively cope with our stress.

Coping with the Emotions

After learning of your HIV diagnosis, the typical response would be one of shock, disbelief, fear, and sadness. Fortunately, these feelings do resolve in time. An emotional reaction to a new HIV diagnosis is expected and should be allowed to play itself out. There are methods the HIV-positive person can use to better cope with the emotional aspects of an HIV diagnosis. These methods include:

- Share your feelings with family, loved ones, your doctor, or a professional counselor. Keep in mind that in order to share your feelings, you will most likely have to disclose your HIV diagnosis. And as we learned earlier, disclosure adds significantly to an already emotional situation. Disclosure can be difficult, but it can be done. Review Chapter 4 to learn how to disclose your diagnosis with the least amount of stress possible.
- Find an effective means to relieve your stress, such as exercising, swimming, or finding a hobby. Find and join a support group in order to share your experiences with people experiencing the same emotions. Support groups make it possible for you to learn ways to deal with your emotions from people who have been there already. As the saying goes, "There's strength in numbers." Support groups help you take advantage of that strength and illustrates that you are not alone in your fight against HIV.
- Get plenty of rest each night, allowing your body and mind to rest and recharge. Adequate rest is essential to a physical and emotional recovery. Learn and employ relaxation techniques, such as meditation and deep breathing exercises, to assist with sleep issues. Because caffeine and nicotine are stimulants, limit the amount you ingest, especially before going to bed.

Dealing with the emotional aspects of HIV is very difficult. Even the most emotionally strong person will eventually need some sort of emotional support, if only for a short period of time. The easiest way to find the support you need is through support groups. Support groups are comprised of people from all walks of life who share a common illness. This commonality works in favor of the group's members, each learning from the experiences of others within the group. These groups can be found in medical practices, community agencies, churches, schools or anywhere there are HIV-infected people coming together to help one another. Let's look a little closer at support groups and what to look for when trying to find a group that is right for you.

Support Groups

In many ways, HIV is like any other chronic disease. The emotional impact of chronic illnesses can be devastating — many times as devastating as the physical effects of the illness. Feelings of fear, anger, and isolation are commonly felt by people with chronic disease. However, for all the similarities, in many ways HIV is unlike any other disease. As an example of how HIV differs, let's look at another chronic illness— diabetes. When a person learns they have diabetes, there will be feelings of fear, anger, and isolation. But in the case of diabetes, the person living with diabetes seldom has to face these feelings alone. When a person is diagnosed with diabetes, people gather around to offer love and support in any way they can. The person with diabetes doesn't have to worry about being labeled or stereotyped because they have diabetes. Prejudice is seldom predicated on the basis of a person's blood sugar. However, when a person is diagnosed with HIV, people tend to move away, unable or unwilling to offer support. Many times the newly-diagnosed are on their own until family and loved ones deal with their own feelings surrounding the new diagnosis.

Support groups provide HIV-positive people with the emotional support they so desperately need. Support groups can also be a benefit to loved ones, caregivers, and family of the HIV-positive person as well. These groups provide a safe, non-judgmental atmosphere in which HIV-positive people and their family and friends can discuss feelings, concerns, and fears surrounding an HIV diagnosis. Support groups are generally relaxed and informal, which encourages participation of the members. For people dealing with the emotional aspects of HIV, there's no better way for them to realize that they are not alone. Support groups bring together people who are experiencing the same difficult situations to encourage sharing and mutual support of one another. HIV support groups can be open to a variety of people or just to specific groups. For instance, there are groups that allow anyone HIV-infected to join: women, men, gay, or straight. There are also groups that are only open to specific groups of people: HIV-positive women, teens, gay men. Still other groups are for HIV-affected people: those people who are HIV-negative but are impacted by the disease. Members of this type of group can include loved ones, caregivers, and medical professionals. Support groups provide a place where people can interact with their peers to discuss the impact HIV has on their life.

Support groups can be especially beneficial for the HIV-infected person. As illustrated earlier in this chapter, people are often alone in those first days after learning of their HIV diagnosis. Support groups offer a place of acceptance amid a world of rejection and prejudice. So many emotions confront the newly-diagnosed and those around them. Changing medical, social, and financial situations cause fear and worry; rejection and prejudice cause depression, anger, and isolation. Support groups can help cope with all those feelings.

Countless studies have demonstrated the benefits of a support group for people infected with and affected by HIV. One study showed that 86 percent of people who attended an HIV support group showed dramatic improvement in how they handled the stress of the disease. It's also been shown that people attending HIV support groups showed more improvement in their depression symptoms when compared to standard psychotherapy sessions. Finally, evidence suggests that members of HIV support groups make better choices with regards to safer sex practices than those who don't attend peer-type support groups. Brett Grodeck, author of the book *The First Year — HIV: An Essential Guide for the Newly Diagnosed*, summed up the benefits of support groups in one sentence: "Talking with other people in similar situations can help you come to terms with your own situation."

SUPPORT GROUP TYPES

Support groups can typically be place into one of four types. They are typed according to how they are conducted. In other words, does the support group have specific rules, guidelines, structure, and a leader? Let's look at the four types.

- *Structured Format* — These groups feature a very structured, almost ritualistic format, following written guidelines and rotating facilitators (facilitators being the person who leads the group).
- *Free Form* — These groups can have rotating facilitators or no facilitator at all. If there is a format, it's very loose, allowing the meeting to progress in a free-flowing manner without having to adhere to a structured format.
- *Trained Volunteers* — These groups are led by people who donate their time and are trained in the proper way to facilitate support groups. These groups usually have written agreements and ground rules on how group sessions will be conducted. Members agree in writing as to what can be discussed and how the meetings run each session.
- *Professional Facilitators* — The guidelines and format of this type of group varies according to the style of the professional who is facilitating the group. These facilitators are typically trained, professional counselors, social workers, or health care professionals.

THE ROLE OF THE FACILITATOR

Most support groups do have a facilitator that guides the activity of the group. Some facilitators are members of the group, while others are paid or volunteer to be an outside observer and leader. The facilitator performs many roles for the group, including:

- working to make sure the group operates effectively and according to written guidelines and formats,

- assuring that discussions adhere to written rules and approved topics,
- setting meeting boundaries and determining topics to be discussed.

Many times there will be co-facilitators in a group. This could be a male and female, a nurse and social worker, or HIV-positive and -negative facilitators. Studies have found that co-facilitated groups are very effective due to their providing two perspectives and two areas of expertise.

FINDING A SUPPORT GROUP

One look at the Internet will tell you there are literally hundreds of support groups to choose from. But like a kid in a candy store, having such a large number of choices can make it more difficult to find what you are looking for. But there are proven ways to find the group that is right for you.

- Speak with your HIV specialist, nurse, or social worker to see if one of them can recommend an HIV support group in your area.
- If you're seeing a psychiatrist, counselor, or psychologist, ask if they can recommend a support group and the characteristics you should look for in a support group.
- Use the Internet to search for support groups in your area. Make certain you are using reputable websites when looking for information.
- Speak with the community-based organizations in your area. It's possible that one of the local HIV agencies will offer a support group as part of their services. If not, they should be able to direct you to an agency that does.

CHARACTERISTICS OF A GOOD SUPPORT GROUP

Different people are looking for different things from a support group. Are the group meetings nearby? Can family members attend group sessions with me? Is there child care available while the group meets? What makes a support group beneficial is very individualized and varies from person to person. But there are characteristics that all support groups should have. These include:

- The group should have regularly scheduled meetings in a safe, easily accessible location (e.g., the location should be on a bus route).
- The support group should have access to mental health and medical professionals that are willing to participate in the support group from time to time. The best way to find these types of support groups is through hospitals or mental health practices in your community.
- The group should have a clearly defined confidentiality policy, and members should have to sign confidentiality agreements if necessary.

THINGS TO KEEP IN MIND

So now you know what traits your support group should have. What other factors should you keep in mind when choosing an HIV support group?

- What do you hope to get out of the support group? Do you want medical information? Are you looking for peer interactions? Are you looking for emotional support?
- Do you want a group run by professionals or by its members?
- How far from your home is the support group located?
- Is there child care available during meeting times?
- Who is allowed to attend support group meetings with you?

Relationship Issues

Life is meant to be shared with someone you love. But the first step in love is dating — looking to find that special someone to share your life with. One of the most common myths surrounding HIV is that, once diagnosed, you must give up any chance of meeting your special someone and give up on the dream of having a family. In fact, I hear from newly-diagnosed people every day telling me they intend to give up dating for good. That doesn't need to happen. With the right precautions and a lot of honesty, people living with HIV can date, have sexual relationships, and find that special someone to share their life. Let's look at dating and the potential issues that arise when living with HIV.

DATING WITH HIV

In Chapter 4 we discussed HIV disclosure. To review, the law requires that any potential sexual partner be made aware of your HIV status before any sexual contact occurs. Is there a perfect time to disclose your HIV status? Probably not. Disclosing your HIV status is frightening whenever you choose to do so. In fact, it may be the hardest thing you'll ever have to do. But what if your relationship hasn't reached that sexual stage? What if sex has yet to enter the picture? Some fear disclosing too early in a relationship will end the relationship and at the same time jeopardize confidentiality for no reason. Others fear that disclosing late in the relationship will be perceived as dishonest. There are two schools of thought regarding when HIV disclosure should take place.

- **Kiss and Tell** — These people choose to "kiss and tell," meaning they will go on a few dates before disclosing their HIV status. This does have its advantages. It allows you to wait and see if the relationship is going to get serious before disclosing. If the relationship stalls, your status was not disclosed needlessly. In other words, people who "kiss and tell" feel this option limits the number of people who become aware of their diagnosis, preserving confidentiality.

• ***Tell and Kiss*** — These people choose to "tell and kiss," meaning that disclosure occurs very early in the relationship, in some cases on the first date. Early disclosure occurs at a time of very little emotional attachment between the two people. It's a fact of life that some people will not be ready or willing to date an HIV-positive person. For many, it's less painful to be rejected early in the relationship before any emotional attachment has occurred. An added benefit of early disclosure is the honesty it implies. Delaying disclosure may be viewed by some as dishonest, as if you are trying to hide something that could have a very significant impact on the relationship. A final consideration regarding early disclosure is what it says about the relationship in general. If you disclose early and the relationship succeeds, you know that success has a foundation in honesty. You can take comfort in knowing that your new partner, girlfriend, or boyfriend accepts you and your diagnosis.

Regardless of when you choose to disclose, it can't be emphasized enough that disclosure must take place prior to any sexual contact — oral, anal, or vaginal.

DATING TIPS FOR HIV-POSITIVE PEOPLE

It goes without saying that the first time you date after being diagnosed with HIV is going to be a very stressful and frightening experience. There are a few things to keep in mind that may just make the situation much easier for you and your prospective partner.

• Some find it easier to date only HIV-infected people. If this is your choice, there are HIV-positive dating services on the Internet that can be helpful. Keep in mind that many social networking sites are primarily used for anonymous sexual "hook-ups." These types of encounters carry considerable risk of exposure to sexually transmitted diseases, including HIV. Some people consider taking personal ads in publications targeted at HIV-positive people, or at groups with a high incidence of HIV, such as the gay population. It's important to note that dating solely HIV-positive people does not imply that safer sex is unnecessary. Because of the risk of sexually transmitted diseases such as chlamydia and gonorrhea as well as the risk of HIV re-infection (see chapter 2), safer sex and condoms are a must with each and every sexual encounter even between two HIV positive people.

• Talk to other HIV positive people who have resumed dating. Ask how they disclosed their diagnosis, what the experience was like, and if they have any advice for someone entering the dating world for the first time since being diagnosed with HIV.

- Be prepared for a reaction after you disclose. It is hard to predict what that reaction will be, as it can range from supportive understanding to rejection and abandonment. Rest assured there will be a reaction, so be prepared and keep in mind the reaction may not be what you are hoping for at that time.

- Before disclosing your status, assess the relationship and the person you are about to disclose to. What will you gain from disclosing? Is the relationship worth risking your confidentiality? Again, keep in mind that disclosure is required regardless of your assessment of the relationship if sex is going to occur or may occur.

- Be prepared for rejection, being let down, and feeling discouraged. With that being said, don't be afraid to get your feet wet. Nothing ventured, nothing gained.

- HIV does not define who you are or what type of person you are. HIV does not rob you of your desires, your goals, or your personality. Healthy, rewarding relationships are possible for people living with HIV. Don't compromise your standards or settle for anyone less than you desire for fear of that person being your only choice. HIV does not mean you are desperate. Don't let the disease rob you of your self-esteem.

- If you choose to use online services to find a date, use the same precautions anyone using such services would use. Your first meeting should be in a public place. Do not divulge too much personal information too soon. Do not let your guard down until you are sure the person you have met online can be trusted and are who they claim to be.

So that date you had led to a second date, then to a third. Before you know it, the two of you are a couple in a full-fledged relationship. Sounds like the perfect scenario, doesn't it? It can be, but there are situations that can stress any relationship. One type of relationship that offers unique challenges is the relationship comprised of one HIV-positive member and one HIV-negative member. These types of relationships are called *serodiscordant*.

The Cause of Stress in Serodiscordant Relationships

In an age when HIV-positive people are becoming more readily accepted by those around them, relationships that include one HIV-negative and one HIV-positive partner are becoming more common. One would be safe in saying that serodiscordant relationships can be riddled with anxiety, fear, confrontation, and a great deal of stress. One would think that in a relationship where a partner is HIV-positive, the cause of stress would be obvious. However, there are reasons for stress that you may not have thought about.

Transmission vs. Care Giving

In couples with two HIV-negative partners, the goal of both partners is the same: to stay HIV negative. However, in couples with one HIV-negative partner and one HIV-positive partner the goal or focus of each partner is different. The positive partner is concerned about transmitting the virus to the negative partner. In other words, the goal is to keep the negative partner HIV-free. The negative partner, on the other hand, devotes his or her attention to their positive partner's health. In other words, they become the care-giver in the relationship. Or, simply put, the goal is to keep the positive partner healthy. This small difference in perspective, goal, and focus causes emotional conflict within the relationship, ultimately increasing the level of stress and anxiety.

How Did This Happen?

If one partner becomes positive while in a relationship, the first question the other partner will ask is, "How did this happen?" If the new infection is the result of unprotected sex outside the relationship, or a consequence of sharing needles while injecting drugs, chances are the negative partner had no idea either behavior was occurring. The stress caused by the new HIV infection is compounded by feelings of anger, betrayal, and sadness as the reality of their partner's infidelity and drug use sets in.

Overly Cautious

In any serodiscordant relationship, there is concern and fear at the prospect of spreading HIV to the negative partner. Because of fear, the couple may become overly cautious in their sexual relationship, putting an end to any sexual or intimate contact for fear of spreading the infection. While it's not the most important part, sexual intimacy is an essential aspect of any loving relationship. Without intimacy, feelings of frustration, longing, and resentment will surface, and, as a result, the relationship will suffer.

Survivor's Guilt

Guilt can be a powerful but destructive emotion. Typically, survivor's guilt is a product of a traumatic event, such as a car accident, in which one person survives while many others die. The sole survivor feels guilty for having lived while so many others died. In a serodiscordant relationship the negative partner feels guilty for being healthy while his or her partner is living with HIV. The guilt becomes more intense if the positive partner has medical issues or becomes sick as a result of their HIV. In extreme cases, the negative partner wishes to be HIV-infected, feeling that being infected would relieve the guilt and, with it, the stressors related to that guilt.

The Desire to Have Children

Most couples in a loving, committed relationship will consider having a family at one time or another. The decision to start a family is a stressful one for any couple. But the concerns of a serodiscordant couple are unique. Obviously, outside of artificial means, unsafe sex is the primary way couples try to get pregnant. And as we all know, unsafe sex carries a considerable HIV risk for the negative partner. This, compounded with concerns over the HIV risk to the unborn child, creates a very stressful atmosphere at a time when couples should be enjoying the realization that they are going to be parents.

Keep in mind that ninety percent of the issues that strain a serodiscordant relationship are no different than those in any other relationship. However, it's the other 10 percent that is the most challenging. What are those issues unique to the serodiscordant couple?

ISSUES FACING SERODISCORDANT COUPLES

Money / Employment

Money problems affect most any relationship at one time or another. But when it comes to serodiscordant relationships, the cause of money problems can be unique. The cost of HIV care and HIV medications is astronomical. Staying health requires regular trips to your doctor, sometimes once each month or even more frequently. These visits can be very time consuming and can limit the number of hours that can be worked. As we all know, time is money, and while you can't put a price tag on your good health, the fact of the matter is that when you are at the doctor you're not working, and if you're not working your income will decrease accordingly. And depending on the health of the individual, holding down a regular, full-time job can be extremely difficult. As money becomes scarce, unpaid bills, credit card balances, and late mortgage payments can accumulate, adding even more stress and anxiety to the relationship.

All the stress and anxiety related to financial difficulties can lead to resentment from the healthy partner. He or she can begin to question their partner's contributions to the household finances. Questions like "Why am I doing all the work?" can surface at some point. On the other hand, it's not uncommon for the positive partner to harbor a tremendous amount of guilt when he or she is unable to pull their share of the financial weight. Along with the guilt, the positive partner can become angry and resentful, realizing that their HIV infection is the primary reason the couple is having financial difficulties.

To Disclose or Not to Disclose

Disclosure is stressful. That much we know. But it becomes a source of relationship stress when each partner has a different idea of who should be told about the HIV infection and who shouldn't. In this situation, one rule applies to every couple: except in circumstances of medical emergency or medical necessity, who is to be told about the HIV infection and when they are told is at the sole discretion of the positive partner. If the positive partner says no to disclosure, then the negative partner must abide by his or her wishes without question. The negative partner should never make independent decisions regarding disclosure.

Sharing Medical Information

Some positive people want their partner with them at every doctor's visit. Other positive people prefer to keep the medical part of their life private. At times, some negative partners have a hard time understanding this. It's natural for people in a committed relationship to want to be included in all aspects of their loved one's life, including medical issues. Leaving a loved one out of medical decisions spawns fear and doubt, two emotions that will undermine any relationship. Some people see that reluctance to share medical information as dishonest and an attempt to harbor secrets. Eventually these feelings will fester into major relationship issues.

Differences of Sexual Comfort and Desire

In a serodiscordant relationship there will be differing opinions regarding sex and intimacy. How much exposure risk is each partner willing to take? What type of safer sex practices will be used? In what sexual activities is each partner willing to participate? A good rule of thumb is that if either partner does not want to engage in an activity or take a risk with unsafe sex, then that partner has the final say. Regardless, differences in sexual drive and risk-taking can become divisive in a serodiscordant relationship.

Fear of the Future

As is the case with any person living with a chronic illness, there is a significant amount of fear and uncertainty surrounding the future. The positive partner is uneasy, fearing the prospect of deteriorating health and an uncertain future. The negative partner dwells on questions such as *"How long will my loved one be healthy?"* or *"How long will he or she be alive?"* Fortunately, advances in HIV care has resulted in promising futures and normal life spans for the HIV-positive person. As people continue to live longer and healthier, couples will become more optimistic about what their future holds. Until then, the concept of an uncertain future will continue to cause a great deal of stress and anxiety in the serodiscordant relationship.

DEALING WITH STRUGGLES—MAKING IT WORK

For as many barriers and issues that exist in serodiscordant relationships, they can be fulfilling and can work. The fact of the matter is that, like any relationship, it takes work and commitment from both partners. Psychologist

Robert Remien of the HIV Center for Clinical and Behavioral Studies in New York City has done extensive research on the issues facing serodiscordant couples. He reminds us all that there are ways to work through the rough spots and enjoy the good ones. Here are a few ideas.

- Never stop talking to one another about the relationship issues that arise. Share your feelings, regardless of how sensitive or painful it may be. While the pain is short term, the benefits from openly discussing issues will have lasting effects for the relationship.
- Consider seeking professional counseling whenever issues arise that can't be worked out alone. Whether it's individual counseling, couples counseling, or both, it can be beneficial to have an impartial, trained eye to help you through the tough times.
- Keep issues in perspective. Obviously, the difference in your HIV status is significant. After all, one of you is positive and one is negative. But that difference should not define your relationship. It's only one of many characteristics that define you as a couple and as individuals. Celebrate the things you have in common and those differences that add to the relationship.
- Take care of one another. All relationships need partners who are willing to care for one another, treat one another with respect, and show the loving emotions that brought you together in the first place.
- Remember that you love one another. There is a reason you are together in the first place. Never be afraid to remind one another now and again. Small little reminders of the feelings you have can do wonders to get you through a stressful time in the relationship.
- Be realistic about your situation. Don't fool yourself into thinking the difference in your HIV status will not affect the relationship in some way. There will be times that one partner or the other will feel like they can't take the stress any longer. Don't fake it; if you are unhappy, say so.
- Stay safe and create sexual guidelines that you can both live with. Plan to discover new ways of eroticizing your lovemaking. Make it fun, laugh more, and don't be so serious. Share any fears, concerns, or feelings you may have related to sexual activities. The key to a successful relationship is to be open and honest.

We have talked about the physical and emotional aspects of HIV and AIDS. It should be clear to you now that HIV indeed impacts the entire person, and it should be treated with that in mind. So, naturally, if HIV affects the whole person, the best way to stay healthy and live with HIV is to make healthy lifestyle choices that affect the entire person.

The following chapters look at lifestyle choices, both healthy and not so healthy. Let's start with an unhealthy choice — substance use and abuse.

11

Substance Use and Abuse

As you have just learned, this text devotes an entire chapter to the psychosocial aspects of HIV. That should illustrate the significant impact HIV has on the emotional health of HIV-positive people. Since early on in the epidemic, experts have recognized the effect HIV has on the entire person — emotional as well as physical. In fact, many feel the psychosocial effects of HIV can be as detrimental as the physical aspects of the disease. Different people handle the emotional aspects of HIV in different ways. Some turn to support groups in an effort to deal with the psychosocial stresses of HIV. Others engage in individual counseling to help adjust to their new diagnosis. And others turn to family and loved ones to receive the emotional help they need. But, sadly, there are many people who seek solace in a liquor flask, a pill bottle, or a needle and syringe. It is for these people that this chapter was written.

While substance use can be a means by which HIV-positive people try to cope with their diagnosis, it also contributes significantly to the number of people living with the disease. In fact, since the epidemic began, intravenous drug use (IVDU or IV drug user) has directly or indirectly been responsible for about one-third of all AIDS cases in the United States. Of those AIDS cases related to IVDU, one in every four persons is a member of a minority group, such as African-Americans or Hispanics. It's obvious that substance use plays a very significant role in the spread of HIV — so much so that the Health Resources and Services Administration's HIV/AIDS Bureau (HRSA/HAB) has devoted considerable funds from the Ryan White CARE Act to the treatment of substance abuse and recreational drug use. HRSA/HAB recognized early on in the epidemic that because substance use contributes significantly to the growing number of HIV-infected people, drug treatment would be necessary to keep people healthy and to slow the HIV epidemic. The funds provided by the CARE Act not only support substance abuse treatment but also make it possible for people with substance abuse issues to access HIV care.

Needle Sharing and HIV

We've established the fact that intravenous drug use is a contributing factor to the HIV epidemic. Sterile needles and syringes are seldom available to IVDU. In fact, most states require a prescription to purchase needles and syringes. Because most IVDU have no medical need for their needles and syringes, they are unable to get a prescription to purchase the needle and syringe they need. Unable to get them legally, IVDU will obtain needles and syringes any way they can — most often illegally from very unreliable sources.

Because sterile needles and syringes are so difficult to come by, it's common practice for IVDU to share their needles and syringes with one another. In fact, in drug user circles, not sharing your needles and syringes is viewed as selfish, anti-social behavior. An IVDU who won't share is looked upon in a negative light.

Sharing their injection items or "works," as they are called, exposes all IVDU to blood borne illnesses, including HIV. Droplets of infected blood are pulled into the needle and syringe during the injection process. These droplets are then injected, along with the drug, into someone else, exposing that person to the blood borne illness of the person from whom they "borrowed" the needle and syringe. It's this type of sharing and reuse that drives the HIV epidemic among IVDU.

One obvious solution to the problem of sharing needles is abstinence from injecting drugs. However, kicking a drug addiction is very difficult, even when there is the desire to quit. Most often there is no desire to stop, and without the will to stop, intravenous drug use will continue. At the very least, stopping intravenous drug use requires a long detoxification process, followed by a long period of group and individual counseling. In other words, it requires a long-term commitment.

Having drug users kick the habit would be the ultimate goal of HIV prevention efforts. Think about it; if people don't use drugs, they don't share needles. If they don't share needles, then their HIV risk is reduced dramatically. To an HIV prevention specialist such a scenario would be a perfect solution to the HIV problem that now exists among injection drug users. Unfortunately, a scenario of universal abstinence from the injection of illegal drugs is neither probable nor realistic. So another solution is obviously needed. Needle exchange has proven to be that solution; but, sadly, it's clouded with controversy.

To many, needle exchange is believed to be nothing more than a means for addicts to get what they need in order to inject illegal drugs. Many politicians view needle exchange as a hot button issue that could spell political suicide for anyone publicly supporting the concept. As a result, political support and monetary funding for needle exchange programs is scarce. The situation begs the question: if needle exchange is as effective as studies have shown, why is there so little support from the people who hold the purse strings?

Needle Exchange Programs

The simple fact remains that sterile needles and syringes are not easy to get your hands on if you're an IV drug user. And because they're so hard to come by, IVDU resort to sharing dirty needles in order to satisfy their need for opiates. Even in those rare circumstances where clean needles are available, most IVDU do not have the financial or medical means to get them. The criminalization of drugs and drug paraphernalia make IV drug users reluctant to secure sterile needles and syringes through legal channels. So the only remaining option is to share the few needles and syringes they do have. Because needles and syringes are desperately needed to satisfy the powerful dependence on opiates, refusal to share needles is, ironically, considered bad etiquette among drug users. In fact, refusing to share puts the user at considerable risk for retaliation from other users desperate to get their next opiate fix. Think of it as an extreme case of peer pressure, and usually the user will give in and share.

To combat the problem of needle sharing, and offer drug users a less risky alternative, needle exchange programs have emerged. These programs are based on the concept of risk reduction — if the risk can't be entirely eliminated, then the next best thing is to reduce the risk. Because kicking the opiate habit is unrealistic for many people, the next best thing is to reduce the risk of IV drug use by using only sterile needles to inject drugs.

Needle exchange programs reduce the HIV infection risk by providing sterile needles and syringes in exchange for used ones. Drug users bring their dirty needles and syringes to a needle exchange site and are given a new sterile needle and syringe in return. Not only does this decrease the HIV risk of the person exchanging the needle, but actually decreases a number of people's HIV risk. By taking one needle and syringe out of circulation, the HIV risk for several people has been decreased. That one used needle and syringe potentially could have caused dozens of HIV infections.

Needle exchange programs are most often part of community-based HIV agencies (typically, agencies concerned with HIV testing and prevention, or that offer case management services). To maximize accessibility, these programs are usually mobile — housed in motor homes, buses, or trucks, which makes it possible for the agency to take the needle exchange program into the community where it's needed most. For instance, in large urban areas you may find a needle exchange van parked near food banks, homeless shelters or halfway houses (anywhere IV drug users are known to frequent). Often, drug users are reluctant, unwilling, or unable to go to the HIV agency where the needle exchange program is housed. Therefore, in order for needle exchange to be successful it has to be taken to those hard-to-reach people, which means going into the community where IV drug users frequent.

Typically, the needle exchange program is much more than a place where needles and syringes are exchanged. The agencies that operate these programs take advantage of the time they have with the IV drug user by incorporating other important services into the needle exchange program. It's a concept borrowed from the retail industry. Retail stores will have big sales in order to get buyers into the store. Once in the store, buyers will purchase other items along with the sale item. In the case of needle exchange, the offer of free sterile needles and syringes brings the IV drug user to the needle exchange professionals. Once with the needle exchange staff, the IV drug user is offered other services in addition to the needle exchange. For instance, they can meet with an HIV test counselor, case manager, or addiction counselor. Some programs will make meeting these other professionals mandatory in order to get the sterile needle and syringe. In many cases, medical examinations are also offered in an attempt to get HIV-positive drug users into HIV care if they are not in care already. In essence, the needle exchange program serves a two-fold need: it's a means to decrease needle sharing, and it's a way to reach an otherwise hard to reach population, bringing to them the other services they so desperately need.

However, HIV professionals realize that it's a very fine line between offering additional services and scaring people away from the program altogether. For instance, those people reluctant or afraid to be HIV tested will shy away from a needle exchange program that requires HIV testing as part of the exchange. The services must be presented as a recommended option, not a requirement that will scare people away. But for those IV drug users who are willing, HIV testing, counseling, and medical care are additional benefits available in many needle exchange programs.

Over the years, scientific data has proven that needle exchange is an effective means of decreasing the spread of HIV among IV drug users. So you would assume that governments are eager to fund such programs. After all, it's a simple way to cut HIV infection rates among IV drug users. Unfortunately, it's not that simple. In fact, in the United States politicians and government leaders are very reluctant to support and promote funding for such programs. In fact, it is against the law for the U.S. government to provide funding for needle exchange programs. Why, you ask? The answer is simple. It's politics. The politics of needle exchange is a major barrier to this effective HIV risk reduction method.

THE POLITICS OF NEEDLE EXCHANGE

The truth is that needle exchange has been proven to be an effective HIV risk reducing method. If that's the case, then why are the politicians and government officials holding the purse strings so reluctant to take a stand and provide the funding necessary to make needle exchange programs a reality? One would think people would jump at the chance to slow the HIV rate. After all, common sense tells us that programs proven to be effective in slowing the HIV epidemic should be funded and put in place across the country. Unfortunately, it doesn't seem to be that easy.

The fact of the matter is that needle exchange is a politically charged issue that very few want to take on. It's because of the controversial nature of needle exchange that exchange programs are not being federally funded. In fact, federal law states that it's illegal to use government monies to fund needle exchange programs. And because of political pressure, few government leaders are willing to chance losing their next election in order to change laws preventing government funding of needle exchange. So until the laws change, needle exchange programs must rely on private funding sources and the few state and local funding opportunities that exist. Unfortunately, because these sources are closely tied to changes in the economy, they can be very tenuous and short-lived, and ideally shouldn't be relied upon to keep programs afloat for long periods of time.

THE ARGUMENT SUPPORTING NEEDLE EXCHANGE FUNDING

Proponents cite several reasons why needle exchange laws preventing government funding should be repealed:

- Data shows that nine out of every ten cases of heterosexually transmitted HIV are related to IV drug use and sharing needles.
- HIV surveillance data shows that around the world, HIV transmission increases in areas where needle sharing and injection drug use is common.
- Numerous studies have demonstrated that needle exchange programs contribute to decreased rates of HIV transmission rates among IV drug users.
- Studies have concluded that needle exchange does not increase the probability that a person will start using injection drugs.
- Finally, studies have shown that the number of people entering drug treatment programs increases in the presence of needle exchange programs.

THE ARGUMENT AGAINST NEEDLE EXCHANGE FUNDING

Opponents of needle exchange are quick to point out dozens of reasons why they feel funding needle exchange is a mistake. Opponents have expressed many concerns. According to opponents:

- Funding needle exchange sends the "wrong message" to children. Opponents are concerned that the concept of needle exchange conveys to children and young people that IV drug use is an acceptable behavior with few consequences.
- Needle exchange enables IV drug use, especially among those populations already ravaged by drug addiction. Opponents believe that removing a barrier to IV drug use will result in more people injecting drugs. In turn, if

more people inject drugs, it follows that more people will become HIV-infected.

- The practice of needle exchange is in stark contrast to the U.S. government's fight against drugs. The government's commitment to reducing drug use includes decreasing the number of needles and syringes on the streets. Any federal funding of needle exchange will increase their numbers on the street — a practice that would contradict the government's stance on drug use.
- If needle exchange programs are funded by the government, it means your tax dollars would be funding an illegal activity — in this instance, injection drug use. Few officials are willing to have their name associated with such a practice.
- Distributing drug paraphernalia in the form of needles and syringes is in stark contrast to the accepted morals of our society. These morals say that drug use is bad, and no one, including the federal government, shall do anything to make it easier for people to engage in the activity.
- According to opponents, needle exchange promotes risky behavior and undermines efforts to stem the problems of substance abuse and HIV infection among IV drug users.

WHERE DO WE STAND

Despite efforts from needle exchange supporters, government funding of such programs is not possible. What little government funding of needle exchange does exists is strictly at the state and local level. The majority of needle exchange funding comes from the private sector through fundraising and donations. The state and local governments that do fund needle exchange are severely limited by tightening budgets, worsening economies, and fewer funding dollars, meaning there are no guarantees that the funding will remain. Ironically, the seat of the United States government, Washington, D.C. has decided to fund needle exchange, while the United States government itself continues to deny funding of any sort.

Understanding Substance Use and Addiction

Substance abuse continues to be a major public health issue in the U.S. and around the world. When people talk of addiction and abuse, typically they're referring to illegal drugs such as cocaine, heroin, or methamphetamine. But the fact of the matter is that prescription drug abuse and addiction is as much a problem as is addiction to illegal drugs. The facts bear this out. In a 2005 survey, more than 6 million Americans reported using prescription drugs in the previous month for nonmedicinal purposes. That number exceeds the number of people who abuse heroin, crack, hallucinogens, and inhalants combined.

Addiction and abuse do not necessarily refer to illegal substances. Alcohol, for instance, is a legal substance available at any carry-out. Yet people around the world abuse the drug and fight one of the hardest addictions to beat. The World Health Organization (WHO) estimates that more than 170 million people worldwide suffer from alcohol addiction. Unlike cocaine, heroin, and crystal meth, alcohol is legal and readily available to anyone who wants it, making addiction more likely. Don't let the legality of alcohol fool you into believing its addiction and abuse are less dangerous than illegal drugs. Alcohol addiction is as devastating to the individual and those he loves as any illegal substance. And the sad fact is that of the 140 million people struggling with alcohol addiction, an estimated 78 percent of those people go untreated.

Substance abuse and addiction are not limited to alcohol and drugs alone. In fact, there are addictions all around. For instance, according to a recent survey, nearly 42 million people say they smoke cigarettes every day. Smokers become addicted to the nicotine they take in with each puff. Or there is the research being done at Johns Hopkins. They report that caffeine, the substance found in coffee, soft drinks, energy drinks, and tea, is the most abused drug in the world. Amazingly, in North America alone, 80 to 90 percent of all adults and children consume caffeine on a daily basis. And finally, people even have addiction issues with food. *Compulsive eating* (over-eating), *anorexia nervosa* (starving one's self), and *bulimia nervosa* (binging and purging) are all types and degrees of food addiction. It's obvious from these examples that addiction is a very powerful disease that can touch even the most basic aspects of our life. Let's look at addiction and why it occurs.

The Science of Addiction

The concept of addiction can be a very confusing one. Terms like addiction and dependence are used interchangeably, and, in fact, often are used incorrectly. The misuse of these terms can cloud our understanding of addiction and dependence. In order to fully understand substance abuse we have to understand the difference between drug dependence and drug addiction.

PHYSICAL DEPENDENCE

Defined as the adaptation by the body to a substance to such an extent that when that substance is absent, the body experiences physical withdrawal symptoms. Physical symptoms such as tremors, anxiety, and acute pain result when the body is deprived of the dependent substance. While these symptoms can be very unpleasant at times, they do not confer addiction to a substance.

The key point to remember is that you can be physically dependent on a substance and experience withdrawal symptoms when deprived of that substance and yet not be addicted to that substance.

PSYCHOLOGICAL DEPENDENCE

Defined as the compulsion to use a substance for its pleasurable effects. This can last far longer than physical dependence — weeks, months, years or, in some cases, a lifetime. It's related more to the person's habits and lifestyle than it is to the substance itself. It's rooted in memories of pleasure associated with the substance. People long for those memories, and their drug is merely the means by which their longing is fulfilled. Think of it in another way. Psychological dependence is a "craving" that is psychologically based, as opposed to the physical feelings of withdrawal that accompany physical dependence.

TABLE 10

Physical Dependence
- Defined as the adaptation by the body to a substance to such an extent that when that substance is absent, the body experiences physical withdrawal symptoms.
- Physical symptoms such as tremors, anxiety, and acute pain result when the body is deprived of the dependent substance.
- Physical dependence does not confer addiction.
- You can be physically dependant and not be addicted.

Psychological Dependence
- Defined as the compulsion to use a substance for its pleasurable effects.
- Lasts far longer than physical dependence — weeks, months, years or, in some cases, a lifetime.
- Rooted in memories of pleasure associated with the substance.
- A craving that is psychologically based, as opposed the physical feelings of withdrawal that accompany physical dependence.

ADDICTION

Defined as a behavioral syndrome that's characterized by repeated, compulsive use of a substance or substances, despite adverse physical, psychological, and social consequences. Addiction and the probability a person will become addicted is dependent upon genetic, psychological, environmental, and social factors. This serious condition is typically characterized by diminishing effectiveness of the drug. In other words, addiction produces the need for increasing amounts of a substance to achieve the same affect. For instance, if you once achieved the desired "high" from two tablets of Vicodin, as your addiction progresses it will take three or four tablets to achieve that same "high."

Despite our explanation, understanding the difference between addiction and dependence can be very difficult. Try to think of it this way. Addiction is a behavioral syndrome in which drug use and procurement dominates a person's normal motivation. The user devotes all their energy to finding that next dose of medication. In fact, the addicted person ignores negative social consequences associated with their drug use in order to get more medication. Many will resort to criminal actions, such as stealing, in order to get more drug. But despite the overwhelming power of drug addiction, the user may not or may experience the physical symptoms of withdrawal commonly experienced in physical dependence.

Our Reward System

The human brain is an amazing organ, controlling millions of physiological processes every second. Over the course of evolution, our brains have developed specialized systems that ensure the survival of the human species. One such system involves "rewards" for those behaviors the body believes are essential and must be perpetuated for survival. Activation of this reward system produces changes in mood, affect, and motivation in such a way that the body repeats the behavior in hopes of getting the reward again. These changes can range from a slight mood elevation to intense pleasure and euphoria. In response to these "rewards," the body will direct behavior in hopes of being rewarded once again. As a result, this system assures that behaviors essential for survival are repeated over and over.

The essence of the body's reward system rests in specialized cells deep within the brain. When these cells are stimulated they trigger the release of a specialized substance known as *dopamine.* Dopamine is a *neurotransmitter* — a special chemical that transmits nerve impulses from cell to cell within the brain. There are specialized receptors in the brain waiting to be "filled" by dopamine. When these receptors are filled, mood is elevated and feelings of euphoria flood the brain. The euphoria experienced with the release of dopamine is the brain's reward for the body's essential behaviors. Like giving your dog a treat when he sits on command, your brain treats your body when you engage in a behavior the brain recognizes as important and necessary for survival.

To simplify the concept of a reward system, think of the dopamine receptor as a lock, and dopamine as the key. The only way to unlock the lock is to have they key. Once the key is in the lock, the lock can be opened. The same is true for the brain's reward system. Once dopamine has attached to its receptor in the brain, the reward system can be unlocked, elevating mood and causing euphoria. And like a dog repeating a behavior that wins him a treat, the body will repeat the behavior that elicits mood elevation and euphoria.

Experts believe the body's reward system may be at the root of drug addiction. A drug's ability to stimulate our reward system gives that drug its potential for abuse and addiction. As we have already discussed, the purpose of our reward system is to reinforce certain behaviors and assure that they are repeated. So it's logical to assume that any drug stimulating our reward system — a reward system that produces euphoria and mood elevation — has the potential for addiction. Each time a drug stimulates the body's reward system in response to a specific behavior, that behavior is reinforced. In the case of addiction, taking your drug of choice and the euphoria that goes along with it is the behavior being reinforced, and one that your brain wants repeated over and over.

The Effects of Drugs on the Brain

Drugs like hydrocodone (Vicodin, Norco, etc.), cocaine, heroin, and other opiates have an unnatural effect on the dopamine receptors in the brain. Prolonged used of opiates can actually change the chemical make-up and physiology of the brain. These drugs affect the amount of dopamine released and the way in which receptors use that dopamine.

Different drugs affect our reward system in different ways. Under normal circumstances, cells of the dopamine system are always active, constantly releasing small amounts of dopamine into the brain. The steady release of dopamine is believed to play a role in mood stability. The introduction of certain drugs into the body affects the cells that stimulate the release of dopamine. For instance, heroin increases the rate at which dopamine is released into the brain, meaning the levels of dopamine in the brain also increase. The increased levels of dopamine cause the mood elevation and euphoria characteristic of heroin use. However, the body will eventually eliminate the heroin from the brain, meaning dopamine levels return to normal and the euphoria and mood elevation subside. But the body "remembers" the pleasant effects of heroin and is very motivated to use heroin again and again.

Cocaine has a somewhat different effect on the dopamine receptors of the brain. Instead of stimulating more dopamine to be released, cocaine slows the elimination of dopamine from the brain. As the body continues to produce dopamine at a normal rate, the cocaine slows its elimination, meaning the amount of dopamine increases. Think of it as a glass being filled with water. If water runs into it at a steady rate but does not empty out, the glass fills with water. Dopamine is produced at a steady rate, but because cocaine has slowed its elimination from the brain, the amount of dopamine rises. Dopamine builds up in the brain, and mood elevation and euphoria result. Once again, the brain "remembers" the effects of cocaine and is very motivated to use the drug again.

After being taken for extended periods of time, drugs such as opiates can change the way the dopamine system works. Repeated or prolonged use of substances that affect the dopamine system actually deplete the amount of dopamine in the body. With less available dopamine, stimuli that normally caused an elevation in mood and motivation no longer do so. In essence, there is no longer enough dopamine for the reward system to function properly. At the same time, the dopamine system becomes more sensitive to drugs like opiates, producing a more intense and pleasurable euphoria. Experts believe that this increased sensitivity contributes significantly to the addiction process.

Why Do People Become Addicted?

We now understand how the body becomes addicted to certain substances. We understand the difference between addiction, physical dependence, and psychological dependence. Now we want to answer the big question: why do people become addicted to substances like cocaine and heroin?

Factors Contributing to Addiction

Genetics

One factor that contributes to the risk of addiction is genetics. Experts have found that certain genes in the human genome can increase the probability a person will have addiction issues. In fact, studies have found that approximately 60 percent of drug addiction is related to genetics. In 2003, scientists concluded the *Human Genome Project*—a project to map the 3 billion gene pairs that make up the human genome. As part of that project, scientists mapped about 400 different genes that influence the probability of addiction.

Environment

Studies have shown that genetics alone do not determine a person's probability of addiction. In other words, just because a person has the genetic markers for addiction doesn't mean that person is doomed to a life of drug abuse. Environmental factors, combined with genetic predisposition, determine the probability of addiction. Three environmental factors play the biggest role.

The Community Domain—A person's connection to the community in which he or she was raised or lives in plays a role in addiction. For instance, in those communities where firearms and drugs are prevalent, the risk of addiction is high. Communities that lack activities or ways for the population to connect to the community have shown the highest prevalence of drug use and addiction.

The Peer Domain—One of the biggest factors when assessing addiction risk is peer pressure. Having friends or associates who are addicted increases a person's risk of addiction. Adolescents are especially influenced by peer pressure and the role peers play when assessing the risk or probability of addiction.

The Family Domain—The family environment, specifically the lack of stability in the family, influences the risk of addiction. For instance, family conflict or addiction within the family can increase the risk of addiction for each family member. When parents struggle with addiction, the children in that family will have an increased risk of addiction. Finally, individuals who live impoverished or are subject to physical or emotional abuse have an increased risk of addiction in an attempt to deal with the physical and emotional pain in their lives.

Mental Illness

It's not uncommon for a person to have a dual diagnosis of mental illness and drug addiction. Experts explain that addiction and mental illness are related to changes in the same region of the brain. The area known as the *amygdala* is involved with the generation of emotions, including fear, anxiety, and happiness. Because mental illnesses, including anxiety disorders, unipolar and bipolar depression, schizophrenia, and other personality disorders, is related to the amygdala as well, addiction and mental illness are common bedfellows. In situations of high stress, tension, loneliness, anxiety, or depression, people often turn to drugs for a short respite. Unfortunately, what starts out as a short-term solution for the trials of everyday life becomes a long-term problem with lifelong consequences.

Addiction Treatment

Despite what many believe, drug addiction is an illness— specifically, an illness seated in the brain and its function. Drug addiction does not imply weakness, immorality, or a lack of self-respect. It's an illness, and being an illness it can be treated. And while treatment is typically long-term and emotionally difficult, it can be successful. But there are some key principles common to all successful treatment programs. These principles include:

- There is not a standard treatment plan applicable to every person. Not all treatment programs will be effective for all individuals. For addiction treatment to be effective, it must be individualized to the person, his or her circumstances, and specifics of their addiction. What's the drug of choice, how much does the person use, and how long have they used are all factors that determine which course of treatment is best for them.
- Treatment needs to be readily available for all who want it, addressing all needs of the individual, not just the addiction issues. In other words, the treatment plan must take a holistic approach, addressing the entire person, not just their drug use.
- An individual's treatment plan must be frequently re-assessed and updated. Drug treatment is not something you can start and forget. The effectiveness of the treatment plan must be constantly assessed and altered to address issues that arise once treatment begins. Successful addiction treatment is a dynamic, ever-changing process.

- Counseling and behavioral therapy are essential parts of any successful treatment program. Remaining in treatment for an adequate amount of time is necessary for the treatment plan to be successful. Long-term abstinence from drug use depends on long-term treatment, complete with emotional as well as physical interventions.

- While the treatment of withdrawal symptoms is important for successful addiction treatment, it alone will do little to resolve the addiction problem. Feeling free of withdrawal symptoms allows a person to concentrate on the root cause of his or her addiction problems. Eliminating withdrawal symptoms alone does not mean the addiction issue has been resolved.

- Treatment of co-existing conditions, such as mental illness, must be part of any effective addiction treatment program. Without a holistic approach, successful addiction treatment is rare.

- Addiction treatment does not have to be voluntary for it to be successful. Whether a person is ordered into treatment, or feels treatment is the only way to save a relationship, job, or family, treatment can be successful without being voluntary. However, once in treatment the person has to be committed to kicking their habit. A half-hearted effort has little chance for success.

Effective Treatment Approaches

Treatment of addiction is generally a three-part procedure: detoxification, addiction treatment, and relapse prevention. The therapeutic process is a combination of medical treatment and behavioral therapy. While these approaches can be used alone, most experts agree that a holistic approach using medical and behavioral modification is the most successful.

DETOXIFICATION

Before any behavioral therapy can begin, the addicted person must be free of the substance he or she misused. The detoxification process can be a very difficult and uncomfortable one. As the drug effects ease, withdrawal symptoms will emerge, a result of empty dopamine receptors. Anxiety, nausea, insomnia, and profuse sweating are just some of the withdrawal symptoms one may experience during the detoxification process. And as you can imagine, those symptoms can be quite severe at times. It's the withdrawal symptoms that most often interfere with the treatment process. As was the case before the person sought treatment, drug-seeking behavior dominates a person's thought processes. As long as there are withdrawal symptoms, addiction treatment failure is a possibility. While a person struggles through withdrawal symptoms there is little time or motivation to be involved in an addiction treatment program.

In recent years medications have been developed that help relieve the symptoms of withdrawal while allowing a person to complete the detoxification process. Without withdrawal symptoms, the person is free to focus on treatment and behavioral therapy. These medications have made it possible for drug-addicted people to get the treatment they need while being relatively free of withdrawal symptoms or drug cravings that make overcoming an addiction so difficult.

Suboxone (Buprenorphine + Naloxone)

This drug has been approved for the treatment of opiate dependence; specifically, it has been approved for office and out-patient use. This is an important step forward because it provides an option for those opiate-addicted people who are unwilling to get involved with in-patient detoxification and treatment programs. It's actually two drugs in one pill, each drug having a very important role.

Buprenorphine — This is the active ingredient in Suboxone. Buprenophine is a partial opioid agonist, meaning it can both activate and block the opiate receptors, depending on the clinical situation. Buprenorphine can produce the effects and side effects of other opiates, but because it is a partial agonist, its maximum effects are less than those of full agonists. At low doses, buprenorphine produces enough opiate effect that people who are addicted can abstain from opiates without withdrawal symptoms. Being free of the unpleasantness of withdrawal and cravings gives the opiate-addicted person the opportunity to detox.

Like all opiates, increasing doses of buprenorphine will produce increased effect — but only to a certain point. Unlike other more addictive opiates, buprenorphine has a "dose ceiling," meaning that the effect of buprenorphine increases with dosage to a certain point. When the ceiling dose is reached, additional dosing in excess of the ceiling dose will not illicit more effect. This characteristic means buprenorphine has a lower risk of overdose, addiction, and side effects when compared to full agonists such as Vicodin that do not have dose ceilings.

Finally, buprenorphine has a prolonged effect on the brain. The drug binds strongly to the brain's dopamine receptors. This means the drug is long-acting and does not leave the dopamine receptors easily. For this reason there is no need for re-dosing, as is the case with other opiates. People who use cocaine or heroin must re-dose frequently to maintain the drug's affect. Re-dosing often leads to accidental overdose, which can be fatal. But because of buprenorphine's long-acting properties, accidental overdose is unlikely.

Naloxone — This drug is an opiate antagonist, meaning it blocks the effects of opiates. When taken correctly, Suboxone is dissolved slowly under the tongue. When taken in this manner, naloxone is not absorbed in sufficient amounts to have any clinical effect. In this case the naloxone is "inert," meaning it doesn't have a therapeutic effect. But because Suboxone is an opiate agonist (a molecule that can trigger an opiate receptor) that can produce euphoria in some people, there will be people who will try to misuse the drug. People do this by crushing and injecting the tablets, or swallowing the tablets whole, similar to what is done with cocaine. So in order to prevent misuse of the Suboxone, naloxone was combined with the buprenorphine. When Suboxone is crushed, injected or swallowed whole, the naloxone is absorbed, blocking the opiate effect of the buprenorphine. In some people the naloxone can actually produce significant withdrawal symptoms. Simply put, naloxone prevents the misuse of Suboxone.

How Suboxone Helps Beat Addiction

So as we just learned, Suboxone is much like an opiate. It can produce euphoric effects similar to that of methadone or hydrocodone. Granted, the effects are less intense and limited, but at the very least, Suboxone can quell the powerful hunger for opiates. If that's the case, than why give Suboxone to someone addicted to opiates? Isn't doing so just feeding the drug addiction? At first glance, that's how it would appear. But actually, the addition of Suboxone to addiction treatment plans has in many cases made it possible for addicts to kick their dangerous habit. Here's how that is accomplished.

- When opiates are taken into the body, they attach to receptors in the brain, causing dopamine release and euphoria.
- Eventually, those opiates vacate the receptors, the euphoria fades and the symptoms of withdrawal begin.
- As more receptors empty, the withdrawal symptoms worsen. At this point, when the withdrawal symptoms are significant, Suboxone therapy can begin. In fact, if Suboxone is started before withdrawal, the buprenorphine suddenly replaces opiates in the dopamine receptors, causing the sudden onset of severe withdrawal.
- As the dose of Suboxone dissolves under the tongue, buprenorphine enters the bloodstream and makes its way to the dopamine receptors previously occupied by opiates. As the receptors fill, withdrawal symptoms begin to fade.
- Buprenorphine attaches firmly to the receptors, blocking other opioids from occupying those receptors. Most opiates have a relatively short duration of action, requiring frequent doses and escalating doses to achieve the same euphoric results. Buprenorphine has a much longer duration of action, meaning its effects do not wear off quickly. Longer action means doses can be given less often, and less medication is required with each dose.
- Because buprenorphine occupies the dopamine receptors, there are few, if any, withdrawal symptoms. Free of withdrawal, drug users can stop taking opiates and start working on the root causes of their addiction.

Suboxone has proven to be a very effective adjunct to addiction treatment. One particular study examined opiate abstinence in people taking buprenorphine, compared to those given a placebo (a pill with no medicinal affect). In a 4-week study, almost 21 percent of those patients taking buprenorphine had an opiate-free urine specimen at the end of 4 weeks. Only about 6 percent of the placebo group had a negative urine screen in the same time frame. In addition, investigators measured opiate cravings using a self-reporting survey. Participants taking the buprenorphine reported about 50 percent fewer cravings by the end of 4 weeks, while those taking the placebo reported no change in their level of craving. Finally, participants were more likely to finish 4 weeks of behavioral therapy when taking buprenorphine, compared to those people not taking the medication. It's obvious from this study that buprenorphine can be a very effective addiction treatment tool that improves both treatment compliance and opiate abstinence.

The Suboxone Treatment Plan

While Suboxone (buprenorphine + naloxone) has been proven to be an effective part of drug rehabilitation and detoxification, it's not as simple as taking a pill a couple of times a day. Suboxone alone is not a cure for drug addiction. Experts agree that stopping opiate use is only the first step in kicking an addiction. Treatment specialists have developed treatment programs that use Suboxone and behavioral therapy. Experts agree that therapy is absolutely essential if the treatment plan is to be successful. With that in mind, the typical Suboxone treatment plan is comprised of five steps.

Intake — It's during this initial phase of the plan that your addiction doctor gets to know you and the extent of your drug use. The doctor will conduct a medical and psychological exam to identify any medical issues or past mental illnesses that may affect your recovery. For instance, because it's not uncommon for recovering addicts to experience symptoms of depression, it's important for the doctor to know if you have been diagnosed with depression in the past.

Depending on the program, you may have an addiction nurse and mental health specialist assigned to your case. They, too, will do assessments in order to better understand your addiction. The nurse will be responsible for administering and monitoring your Suboxone therapy, while the mental health counselor will support you from a psychological perspective.

Your doctor must be certain you are healthy physically. Blood will be drawn to assess organ function, especially that of the liver and kidneys. Excessive drug use puts stress on the body's systems, the liver and kidneys in particular. Most drugs must pass through the liver where chemical changes occur. The liver breaks down the drug into smaller compounds that can be used by the body. The compounds that are not used are excreted by the kidneys.

In the event the liver has been damaged by extensive drug use, alcohol use or some underlying liver disease (e.g. hepatitis C), Suboxone will not be broken down and excreted properly. Over time, the drug will accumulate, eventually reaching toxic levels. Excessive blood levels of any drug, Suboxone included, can cause serious health issues and further damage to the liver.

A urine drug screen will also be a part of your initial work-up. It's not uncommon for people with addiction issues to withhold information regarding drug use. Drug addiction is a powerful illness, causing people to lie, cheat or steal to get their next fix. Addiction professionals know that a person's drug use is not always how the patient portrays it. It's very important that the addiction team has an accurate picture of the patient's drug use. Unidentified drug use by the person in recovery can undermine the entire addiction treatment process. A urine drug screen will help identify drug use not revealed voluntarily by the patient. The screen will identify any drugs or alcohol ingested, and will give the treatment team a rough idea of when it was ingested. As the treatment plan progresses, a urine drug screen can identify those patients who are not adhering to the treatment plan.

Finally, the doctor will ask you questions about your opiate use in order to assess the type, amount, and frequency of your drug use. It's absolutely essential that you be completely honest regarding the drug you use, how much you use, and how often you use. Many drug users try to deceive their treatment team, but addiction professionals have heard just about every lie, excuse, and attempt at deception. Pulling the wool over their eyes, so to speak, would be difficult, and in the long run it will only undermine your efforts to get healthy and drug free.

Induction — This phase of treatment is to transition the addict from his drug of choice to Suboxone. This is not as simple as it sounds. It's more complex than just taking a dose of Suboxone and beginning therapy. It is important to be in mild-to-moderate withdrawal when you take your first dose of Suboxone. If you have high levels of another opioid in your system, Suboxone will compete with the other opioid molecules, knocking them off the receptors. Suboxone replaces those opioid molecules on the receptors, but because Suboxone has less opioid effects than the person's drug of choice, you may go into withdrawal and feel sick. The reason Suboxone is used is to minimize the symptoms of withdrawal. Given too early, Suboxone will cause sudden withdrawal, defeating its purpose altogether.

The first dose will be given under the observation of the treatment team. The Suboxone tablet is placed under the tongue and allowed to dissolve, typically over five to ten minutes. Usually, the withdrawal symptoms begin to ease after about an hour. Depending on how well the first dose suppresses withdrawal symptoms, a second dose may be given.

The key point to remember is that Suboxone must be allowed to dissolve under the tongue to be effective. If it's chewed, crushed or swallowed whole, naloxone becomes bioavailable, knocking opiates and buprenorphine from the opiate receptors, causing sudden withdrawal. When dissolved under the tongue, naloxone is not bioavailable, and much more buprenorphine is absorbed, meaning the Suboxone effectively eases the symptoms of withdrawal.

The induction phase of treatment can last as little as one day or as long as a week. During this time, daily visits to your doctor are not uncommon. Direct-observed dosing, meaning the treatment team observes each dose being taken, is used by many programs during this phase. In these programs the treatment team holds onto the Suboxone, giving the patient just enough doses to get them through the night. Urine drug screens are usually included in these daily visits as well.

Stabilization—During the next phase of treatment the Suboxone dose is adjusted to find the lowest possible dose that totally suppresses withdrawal symptoms. Depending on the individual, this phase can take a week or more. This phase is also the time when patient and doctor discuss treatment options—specifically, the advantages of short-term and long-term Suboxone treatment plans. Most addiction programs have a system in place with requirements that have to be met in order to remain in the program.

For instance, a minimum number of group therapy sessions must be attended each week. The number of sessions required is based on the needs of the individual. In essence, when the patient presents him or herself for outpatient addiction treatment, they are contracting with the program and are bound to the rules of the plan. Addiction programs adhere to their treatment plan, with very few exceptions. If individuals miss required meetings or have difficulty adhering to the plan, the program will take issue. In some cases the addict will be asked to leave the program or change to an in-patient program where personal freedom is very limited and the rules are very strict.

An important decision during this phase is how long to use Suboxone in the treatment plan. Some people use the drug only during the detoxification period, slowly withdrawing and discontinuing it soon after the body is clear of opiates. Others use Suboxone throughout the entire treatment period to diminish the risk of relapse. This maintenance dosing can continue for months or longer in order to reduce the risk of relapse. Keep in mind there is no one right approach. Some people need to stay on Suboxone as a maintenance medication. Others do well discontinuing the drug soon after detoxification has been completed. The key to success, however, is not to discontinue Suboxone too soon. If the Suboxone is discontinued before the addict has the tools to resist the powerful drug cravings characteristic of opiates, the chance of sustained abstinence from opiates is slim.

Maintenance—Suboxone can be used throughout treatment and recovery for those patients who choose. However, it can't be emphasized enough how important it is for substance abuse counseling to continue along with Suboxone. In fact, studies have illustrated without a doubt that Suboxone alone is not an effective way to beat a drug habit. The chance for treatment success is greatly improved by attending professional substance abuse counseling after you have stopped taking opiates. For those who choose, Suboxone can be used throughout the recovery process.

Substance abuse counseling is typically a combination of group and individual counseling. Suboxone will be prescribed at the lowest dose that suppresses withdrawal symptoms and opiate cravings. If necessary, this phase can last months or even a year or more.

People may not realize that, because it's a partial opiate agonist, Suboxone can cause some dependence after long-term use. Withdrawing Suboxone treatment is considered to be less difficult than most other opiates such as Methadone. However, the potential for dependence remains and should be considered by the patient and doctor when deciding upon maintenance dosing (long-term Suboxone) versus medically supervised withdrawal (short-term Suboxone).

Medically Supervised Withdrawal—For those who decide Suboxone maintenance dosing is not for them, the drug must be tapered down slowly in order to avoid uncomfortable withdrawal symptoms. If the drug is stopped abruptly, withdrawal symptoms similar to symptoms experienced at the time of induction will occur. During this phase your doctor will slowly decrease your dose, being careful to do so in a manner that produces the fewest withdrawal symptoms or opiate cravings. The eventual goal of this phase is to stop Suboxone treatment altogether.

This can be a dangerous time for the recovering patient. The addict realizes that all he or she needs to do to relieve withdrawal symptoms is to take a dose of opiate. Without the therapeutic effects of Suboxone, patients will be at the mercy of their opiate cravings and withdrawal symptoms. Hopefully, the patient will have the tools necessary to resist the temptation and remain abstinent. Giving in to the cravings will land the person in relapse, and their attempt at stopping their drug use will fail. For this reason, treatment teams must be aware of their patient's commitment to abstinence and their ability to resist. The Suboxone should not be stopped faster than the patient's ability to resist.

The Role of Counseling

While Suboxone treats the physical issues of recovery, professional counseling is an essential adjunct that treats the emotional aspects of addiction. Experts agree that addiction counseling is essential during and after your Suboxone treatment. Think of it this way. Every morning you wake up with a headache. So you take an aspirin to relieve the pain. You feel much better, but the next morning the headaches are back. The aspirin treated the pain but did nothing to find the cause of the headaches. The same is true for addiction. Suboxone can remove the physical manifestations of addiction — namely, drug cravings and withdrawal. However, Suboxone does nothing to treat the psychological root of the addiction. Just like with our headache example, if you don't find the cause of the addiction, most likely relapse will occur. Believing Suboxone is all that is needed to "cure" addiction is a big mistake that can lead to relapse down the road.

Counseling and group sessions explore the root causes of addiction. Why did drug use become such a dominating force in a person's life? Counseling tries to answer that question. Without the answer there can be no long-term solution. Any treatment not involving counseling and behavioral therapy is destined to fail.

The benefits of group and individual behavioral therapy are two-fold. First, therapy helps find the cause or causes of the drug use. Finding the cause gives treatment a better shot at long-term success. Secondly, behavioral therapy teaches the patient how to deal with those causes. For instance, say a man has a drug problem. In order to cope with the everyday stresses of life, this man has chosen to take opiates. Behavioral therapy could help this man make better choices regarding how to cope with the stress in his life. Simply put, through behavioral therapy, the man is taught better ways to deal with everyday stress. Those tools will also help him resist the powerful drug cravings characteristic of opiate addiction. Behavioral therapy prepares you for the battle to beat addiction and dependence. And while addiction relapse is fairly common, studies have shown that behavioral therapy dramatically improves your chances of successful, long-term recovery from opiate addiction and dependence.

12

Dental Care

The importance of regular medical care has been stressed throughout this text. We've learned thus far how important regular healthcare is to people living with HIV. Segments of your healthcare, such as vaccinations, regular health screenings, and adherence to your HIV medication regimen, seem to take priority among patients and providers alike. Yet, there are other areas that are just as important but seem to be forgotten. In this day of visit quotas and ten-minute appointments, these forgotten aspects of your health take a back seat even among HIV specialists. When time is limited and the waiting room is full, doctors have to prioritize. Unfortunately, certain aspects of your overall health are frankly left up to you. One such area is dental care. While most providers will confirm the importance of good dental care, many assign it a low priority during a medical visit. So, most often, tending to your dental health is left to you and your dentist. The truth of the matter is that dental care plays an extremely important role in the overall health of an HIV-positive person. That being the case, let's take a closer look at dental care in the HIV-positive person.

Dental Health

Good dental health, or, more accurately, good oral health, is an important part of a healthy life. Experts agree that HIV patients must maintain functional oral health in order to receive adequate nutrition. And what is functional oral health? Simply, HIV-positive people must maintain a healthy mouth and healthy teeth in order to eat properly. Conversely, mouth pain or teeth pain interfere with eating, meaning the HIV-positive person will not take in enough calories, vitamins, and nutrients to maintain a healthy diet. Functional oral health simply means maintaining your mouth and teeth so you can eat properly.

Many take their dental health for granted until they are suffering with a toothache or "canker sores" that make eating an adventure in pain and torture. Few realize that besides interfering with the diet, poor oral hygiene can be a breeding ground for fungal, bacterial, and viral infections that can affect the entire body. While this is true for most anyone, people with weakened immune systems, such as people living with HIV and AIDS, are especially at risk. Mouth ulcers, gum disease, and tooth decay are all conditions that can cause serious illness elsewhere in the body if left untreated. Here are some key reasons good oral health is important to the HIV-infected person.

- Poor dental health, including loose, missing, or painful teeth, can severely impact the HIV-positive patient's ability to eat. If the patient is unable to eat, proper nutrition is impossible, and HIV progression is inevitable.
- Health issues in the mouth can be one of the first signs of HIV infection and may identify those people with an increased probability of HIV progression.
- A weakened immune system can be further stressed by poor oral and dental health.
- Mouth ulcers, gum ulcers, and decayed teeth can be portals that allow bacteria and other infectious organisms into the blood stream.
- Regular dental exams will help identify oral health concerns early, allowing for treatment before those problems progress to other, more serious infections.

Finding a Dentist

The first step to good oral health is finding a dentist. While there are dentists virtually everywhere, finding a dentist who is comfortable working with HIV-positive people can be a challenge. HIV makes managing other aspects of your health much more difficult. Keeping your mouth and teeth healthy is more difficult for people living with HIV. Many dentists do not feel comfortable with the complexity that HIV adds to dental care. The result is fewer quality dentists to care for HIV patients.

Granted, finding a dentist to care for HIV patients can be difficult and frustrating. But they are out there; it's just a matter of finding the dentist that's right for you. Here are some tips for finding a quality dentist.

- Talk to the local HIV case management agencies. Many keep contact information for dentists that welcome HIV-positive people. Among the HIV community (patients and care givers), these dentists are referred to as "HIV friendly."
- Seek out recommendations from family, friends, and other HIV-positive people. Word of mouth and personal testimonials are two of the best ways to find a reliable quality dentist.
- If you are moving to a new area, speak with your current dentist. It's possible that he or she may be able to recommend a dentist in your new loca-

tion. Prior to relocating, contact the HIV agencies in your new area to get the names of "HIV friendly" dentists.

• When you do find a dentist you like, make your first visit something simple — a cleaning or a consultation. By doing so you can learn about the dentist and the practice without being under the duress of a painful tooth or complicated dental procedure.

• When assessing a new dentist and dental practice, ask yourself the following questions:

  - Do the dentist and hygienist post their credentials?
  - Does the dentist conduct himself in a professional manner?
  - Does he or she explain procedures clearly?
  - Is the dentist willing to answer your questions?
  - Is the office clean and organized?
  - Does the equipment look in good working order?
  - Does the staff treat you with respect?
  - How much do common procedures cost?
  - Does the dentist accept your insurance, and if not, what kind of financial aid packages to they offer?

• Ask the dentist how many HIV patients they see as part of their practice. HIV is a complex disease. To become proficient in HIV care, a doctor or dentist should care for several HIV patients each year. Treating one or two a year is not enough to stay current with all the changes in HIV care.

• Speak with your dentist regarding his or her goal and philosophy of treatment. The dentist should be equally concerned with the appearance of your teeth and your overall oral health. If one or the other seems more important to your dentist, it may be time for a change.

• Use professional organizations, such as the American Dental Association or the Academy of General Dentistry, to find a board-certified dentist in your area.

Barriers to Proper Dental Care

Despite the importance of regular dental care for the HIV-positive person, there are still considerable barriers to obtaining that care. A study from 2003 reported that the three most common barriers to dental care are cost (30 percent), fear of the dentist (19 percent), and low motivation to go to the dentist (13 percent). Those barriers, and a variety of others, translate into unmet dental needs. In fact, the same study reported 65 percent of HIV patients had unmet dental needs over the previous three years. Let's take a closer look at the barriers to dental care for the HIV-positive patient.

Cost

Like all medical care, it is expensive — so expensive, in fact, that the cost is a deterrent to getting the dental care so important to the overall health of the individual. There is dental insurance, but like medical insurance, it's usually provided through an employer. If the person is unable to work full time because of health concerns, that person will not have access to dental insurance at all. If they are lucky enough to have dental insurance, it is often inadequate to cover the entire cost of the services they need. There are publically funded dental care options, but usually they provide only the most basic services — yearly exams and cleanings, for instance. Some states have dental assistance programs with funding from the Ryan White CARE Act; however, these programs have limited funds and often have to turn away new applicants. Finally, some cities, counties or universities have community dental clinics that offer free or discounted dental care.

Fear

Fear of the dentist is so common there is a medical term for this very real condition. *Dentophobia* is defined as a morbid, irrational fear or aversion to going to the dentist. Whatever you call it and however it is defined, fear of the dentist does get in the way of HIV dental care. Sometimes the fear is rooted in a bad experience at the dentist; to some it's the sound of the drill and the fear of needles. Still others fear the pain that is associated with a trip to the dentist. For HIV patients, they have the additional fear of disclosing their HIV status and the fear of prejudice to deal with.

While dentists are well aware of the fears people have, they have no idea you have such a fear unless you talk to them. While it may be a bit embarrassing, the dentist will understand, will not judge, and will be able to offer you options that will help reduce the fear and make your trip to the dentist much less trying. For many, just getting to know their dentist a little better will help diminish that fear. Think of it this way: facing your fear and getting past it is necessary to maintain your dental health and ultimately your overall health. Have the discussion with your dentist. It is well worth it.

Lack of Motivation

Nothing gets done without motivation, that push we need when our inspiration and enthusiasm dwindles away. Without motivation, achievements would not be achieved and goals would not be attained. And if you are anything like me, you need motivated to go to the dentist. For some, the desire to have clean, healthy teeth is motivation enough to get to the dentist regularly. Others need much more; most often they need pain to motivate them. Like we have all experienced at least once, there is nothing like tooth pain. Tooth pain is a great motivator; but, unfortunately, once you have tooth pain the damage is already done. Without the motivation, a trip to the dentist does not happen for most. So here are five tips to keep you motivated.

- Create a situation where you would be embarrassed not to go to the dentist. You could buddy up with another person who doesn't fear the dentist all that much. You can't say no after watching your buddy get his or her teeth cleaned. Peer pressure is very powerful.
- Make lists of what you need to do, including going to the dentist. Taking a daily inventory of what needs to be done makes not going much harder. And with lists, you get the satisfaction of checking off items when you have completed the task — when you have gone to the dentist.
- The third tip relates to the first: stay in touch with other people. These people will motivate you by the fact they have needs and problems as well. For instance, you could sleep until noon, watch television all afternoon, and eat and go to bed and get absolutely nothing done. But by having a spouse, friend, or child in your day, their needs and problems force you to get off the coach and interact with them, getting your items taken care of as well.
- Join a support group or social group. Like our last tip, having others in your life motivates you to get things done in your life. Also, in support groups people share similar needs and responsibilities; or, simply put, everyone in the group needs a trip to the dentist.
- Get in touch with yourself. In other words, learn your disease, learn the steps to staying healthy, and understand what happens if you don't take those steps. Push yourself and demand that you do something each day to stay healthy. As you succeed, your motivation to continue, including adhering to regular dental care, will increase.

Oral Manifestations of HIV

A study appearing in the *Journal of Dental Research* examined just how many bacteria were present in the mouth. While the numbers vary from person to person and from situation to situation, the study reported over 150 million bacteria are present in the mouth at any given time. If that's the case, is it any wonder that there are so many dental and oral problems in the HIV-positive person.

There are many oral manifestations of HIV. Bacterial infections, fungal infections, and viral infections are just some of the problems that HIV patients encounter. And, sadly, history shows that the vast majority of dental problems in HIV patients goes untreated.

FUNGAL LESIONS

Candidiasis

- Commonly called "thrush," this fungal infection is found on the tongue and oral mucosa.
- It presents as white patches that can be scraped off with a toothbrush or tongue depressor.
- It's typically diagnosed by appearance or by examining a smear under a microscope.
- Candidiasis is treated with anti-fungal medications such has fluconazole or clotrimazole troches.

Histoplasmosis

- While this fungal infection typically occurs in other parts of the body, oral lesions can occur.
- It appears as an ulcer of the oral mucosa.
- Histoplasmosis is diagnosed by biopsy.

VIRAL LESIONS

Herpes Simplex

- One of several types of herpes virus, herpes simplex is typically found in the genital area.
- It appears as fluid-filled vesicles that rupture and crust.
- Symptoms include pain and itching.
- Diagnosis is typically made by culturing the lesions and the fluid contained in the vesicles.
- There is no cure for herpes simplex, but outbreaks can be shortened by using anti-viral medications such as acyclovir or valtrex.

Herpes Zoster

- Another of the herpes virus family, herpes zoster's oral lesions are reactivated varicella zoster (the virus that causes chickenpox).
- Typically, herpes zoster causes fluid-filled vesicles on the skin, but oral lesions do occur.
- Initially, symptoms can mimic tooth pain.
- While skin vesicles rupture and crust, oral lesions form ulcers.
- The lesions of herpes zoster are usually in a linear pattern along nerve tracts.
- Diagnosis is made by appearance and the distribution of the lesions.

- Like other types of herpes virus, there is no cure, but anti-viral medications like acyclovir and valtrex can limit the duration of outbreaks.

Human Papillomavirus (HPV)
- HPV typically causes genital warts but does cause oral lesions at times.
- Oral lesions are found most often in people with HIV.
- The type of HPV that causes oral warts is a bit different than those that cause anogenital warts.
- The oral warts appear as single or multiple nodules that resemble cauliflower.
- Diagnosis is made by biopsy.
- The lesions can be surgically removed, but relapses frequently occur.

Cytomegalovirus (CMV)
- While it is fairly rare, oral lesions from cytomegalovirus (CMV) have been reported.
- They can look much like apthous ulcers, except CMV ulcers look necrotic around the borders, not red.
- CMV ulcers are diagnosed by biopsy.
- CMV ulcers appear in cases of systemic CMV infection; therefore, if they do arise, the patient should be assessed for systemic CMV infection.
- The ulcers will resolve with the medication gancyclovir, used to treat the systemic CMV infection.

Hairy Leukoplakia (HL)
- HL presents as an asymptomatic, corrugated or "hairy" looking white lesion on the lateral aspects of the tongue.
- The lesion is non-movable and is more common in people with lower CD4 counts.
- The presence of HL is indicative of a weakened immune system.
- Past studies indicate that people with HL have a higher probability of progressing to an AIDS diagnosis when compared to people without HL.
- HL can be diagnosed by an experienced clinician simply by appearance, but a definitive diagnosis should be done with biopsy.
- Because HL is asymptomatic, it typically does not require treatment.
- HL has been proven to improve in those patients taking acyclovir for a herpes outbreak.
- Fluconazole can be used in those patients who have "thrush" along with HL.

BACTERIAL LESIONS

Periodontal Disease

Periodontal disease is a chronic inflammatory process, bacterial in nature, affecting the tissue and bone structures supporting the teeth. While periodontal disease can occur in anyone, regardless of HIV status, two particularly damaging types are unique to people with weakened immune systems.

Necrotizing Ulcerative Periodontitis (NUP)—This periodontal disease is considered a marker for severe immune system compromise. Formally known as HIV periodontal disease, NUP is characterized by severe pain and bleeding, with rapid and significant bone and tissue loss. Also characteristic of this serious periodontal disease is premature tooth loss and a foul odor from the mouth. Left untreated, this periodontal condition can cause systemic symptoms as well. Treatment includes debridement of the dead and infected tissue by a dental professional using a solution known as *chlorhexidine gluconate*. Oral antibiotics are also indicated. Finally, pain control is an important key. Without adequate pain control, the person will not be able to eat, meaning their nutritional status will not be conducive to proper healing.

Linear Gingival Erythema (LFE)—LFE is commonly called "red band gingivitis" due to its characteristic red band appearance. The red band appears along the gingival (gum) line and may be accompanied by bleeding and pain. While it can extend to all parts of the gum, it primarily affects the front or anterior portions. Some experts believe there is a connection between LFE and chronic *candida* infections. In fact, the American Academy of Periodontology considers LFE a gingival disease of fungal origin. However, antifungal medications are not the treatment. Instead, plaque debridement by a dentist and twice daily mouth rinses with chlorhexidine is the treatment of choice, along with better oral hygiene at home.

OTHER ORAL MANIFESTATIONS

Apthous Ulcers (Canker Sores)

The cause is not well understood, but many possible causes have been theorized:

- vitamin deficiencies
- faulty immune system
- autoimmune inflammation
- various disease states (HIV included)
- injury to the mouth and gums from brushing or poor fitting dentures
- emotional stress
- hormonal changes in women (outbreaks during menstruation and improvement during pregnancy)

Ulcers are not contagious and are not spread orally from person to person. The frequency of outbreaks can be diminished by avoiding things that may cause gum injury such as rough, sharp food that scratches the gum; vigorous brushing that results in an injury to the gums; spicy and acidic foods.

Treatment of canker sores depends a great deal on the cause. Some examples of treatment include changing to a milder tooth paste; using antibiotic mouth rinses; achieving pain relief from topical numbing agents; taking steroids for severe and recurrent cases; and employing antifungal medications, which can be given if the canker sores are related to a candida infection (thrush).

Xerostomia (Dry Mouth)

Xerostomia, commonly known as dry mouth, is the major source of tooth decay in the HIV-positive person. The condition is a result of changes in the quantity and quality of saliva. There are a number of possible causes. They include:

- side effect of various medications, including some HIV medications;
- changes in salivary gland production and saliva quantity and quality;
- a complication of certain illnesses, infections, and diseases, including HIV and AIDS;
- any condition that causes fluid loss and eventual dehydration, such as vomiting, diarrhea, poor fluid intake, and profound blood loss; a very common side effect of radiation therapy used in the treatment of head and neck cancers; blocked salivary glands or glands that have been removed due to tumor growth.

Changes in saliva production can lead to other illnesses. For instance, because saliva is an important part of tooth decay prevention, xerostomia can lead to more rapid and extensive decay. Saliva is constantly rinsing the mouth of sugars left over from eating. These sugars can settle on teeth, eventually causing tooth decay. Also, saliva has antimicrobial properties, meaning it rids the mouth of harmful bacteria. Without the saliva, the unchecked bacteria can cause severe and rapid tooth decay. Experts believe that the severe tooth decay characteristic of the methamphetamine user is in a large part due to xerostomia.

People with xerostomia have several complaints related to their dry mouth, including:

- difficulty speaking, swallowing, chewing, or wearing dentures;
- sores under and around dentures;
- a painful tongue that sticks to the palate;
- a change in, or the absence of, taste;
- the need to drink increased amounts of water;

- cracking of the lips, tongue, and oral mucosa;
- parotid gland inflammation and swelling.

The treatment of xerostomia is typically accomplished by removing the cause of dry mouth when possible. For instance, if it is a medication or medications causing the issue, substituting that drug with another may be all it takes. Sometimes changing the way you take the medication can alleviate the dry mouth. Dry mouth is sometimes affected by the amount of drug in the blood stream at one time. In these instances, merely splitting the medication into smaller, more frequent doses may be all it takes to relieve the symptoms of dry mouth.

Sometimes the cause of xerostomia is not easily removed. In these cases, stimulating the salivary glands may be the answer. Certain chemicals, such as those containing citric acid, can stimulate the salivary glands to produce saliva. Electrical stimulation using very small electrical impulses have been known to work as well. Finally, medications such as salivary substitutes and oral moisturizers may be of some benefit as well.

Kaposi's sarcoma (KS)

In the beginning of the HIV epidemic, Kaposi's sarcoma, or KS as it is often called, was the face of AIDS. All one has to do is watch the movie *Philadelphia* to understand the impact KS legions had on the HIV-infected person — physically, socially, and emotionally. While the incidence of HIV has decreased dramatically since those early days, KS can still be an oral manifestation of HIV and AIDS.

The typical KS lesion can be nodular ("lumpy"), macular (flat), or raised and ulcerated, appearing primarily but not exclusively on the palate. Their color ranges from red to purple, becoming darker as they age. The presentation of oral KS can range from small, flat red or purple areas along the gingiva to large nodular lesions on the roof of the mouth (the palate). These KS nodular lesions can get so large that they impede swallowing and speech. Often times, KS lesions are accompanied by infections such as thrush, cytomegalovirus (CMV), and a variety of herpes-type viruses.

In some instances, oral KS has a very distinctive appearance, making a presumptive diagnosis possible. However, a definitive diagnosis can only be made via biopsy of the lesions. This is especially important in African-American and other people of color because lesions can be missed or misdiagnosed due to the dark color of the oral mucosa in these people.

Treatment of oral KS lesions can be localized or systemic. In fact, a majority of patients need systemic treatment for their KS.

Localized — as the name suggests, localized KS treatment attacks the lesion itself. Radiation therapy directly to the lesion is the most common treatment. Beam radiation is targeted to the lesion, reducing its size over the course of several treatments. However, radiation therapy to the oral cavity produces many unpleasant side effects, including inflammation and burns to the oral mucosa, as well as an overgrowth of fungal and herpetic infections. For this reason, radiation therapy should be limited to those oral lesions producing symptoms or that are impeding swallowing, eating, or speech. Other types of localized treatment include topical creams that impede KS growth, freezing with liquid nitrogen, or chemotherapy drugs injected directly into the KS lesion. Despite best efforts, re-growth of the KS lesion will often occur after 4 to 6 months post-treatment.

Systemic — This form of treatment is reserved for KS that is rapid growing or life threatening. Similar to cancer, systemic treatment consists of chemotherapy medications given intravenously or, in rare circumstances, orally. Chemotherapy drugs are *cytotoxic*, meaning they kill cells — in this case, the KS cells. Because of their cytotoxic nature, the KS rapidly reduces in size. KS treatment can be a single chemotherapy agent or a combination of two or more. Unfortunately, chemotherapy has many side effects, some of which are very unpleasant. Chemotherapy kills healthy cells as well as KS cells, resulting in things like hair loss, nausea, and abnormally low blood counts. Because of these side effects, chemotherapy is reserved for only the most severe or rapidly growing KS.

Because Kaposi's sarcoma is viral in nature, anti-viral medications are sometimes used to treat the lesions. The antiviral medication *Interferon* is an example of such a medication. Used alone, high doses of Interferon are needed to be effective. However, because toxicity and side effects seem to be dose related, high-dose Interferon causes significant toxicity. In response, experts conducted trials using certain HIV medications in conjunction with Interferon. The result was fewer side effects and toxicities because Interferon can be used in lower doses in the presence of some HIV medications. Caution had to be used, however, because the combination of Interferon and some HIV medications caused side effects and toxicities of their own.

Treatment of KS has variable success. Since the advent of HIV medications, the incidence of KS has gone down and the prognosis has improved. While oral KS is seldom fatal, pain, cosmetic changes and possible airway and esophageal obstruction justify aggressive treatment. Most times, peripheral KS can be successfully treated with radiation, but in the case or oral lesions, severe side effects, such as burns and inflammation to the oral mucosa, makes intravenous chemotherapy the better choice.

Oral Hygiene and Health Maintenance

It has been estimated that upwards of 90 percent of all people living with HIV will present with at least one oral manifestation during the course of their infection. Several studies have demonstrated that 40 to 50 percent of all HIV-infected people have oral fungal, bacterial, or viral infections early in the course of their infection. The ability to differentiate one manifestation from another and manage these manifestations is the key to the overall health of the HIV patient. Maintaining the health of the mouth and teeth is the best way to prevent many of these manifestations. Let's take a look at some oral hygiene and oral health tips.

TREAT YOUR DENTURES TOO

As we have learned, one of the most common oral conditions in the HIV-positive person is candida or thrush. People are very good about taking the medications prescribed to get rid of the thrush. But the one thing they forget is that there may be candida on the surface of their dentures as well. It's important to rid your dentures of this candida to prevent reinfection every time you put them into your mouth. This is best accomplished by cleaning the dentures once a day and soaking them overnight in a 1:1 solution of chlorhexidine (a solution with equal parts water and chlorhexidine). The brand name PerioGard Oral Rinse© is a good example of such a solution.

HIV MEDICATION REGIMENS

We know that HIV medications suppress HIV and therefore help preserve the immune system. But a paper published in 2004 points out that in addition to suppressing the HIV virus, initiation of highly active antiretroviral therapy (HAART) decreases the incidence of the oral manifestations of HIV. But as is the case in HIV suppression, HAART works best when the regimen is adhered to as prescribed.

MAINTAINING GOOD DENTAL HEALTH

Keeping your mouth healthy is a very important part of preventing the oral manifestations of HIV. Luckily, the things the individual can do are relatively easy, and most are inexpensive as well.

Brush Your Teeth Twice a Day

Use either a manual or electric toothbrush, but make sure the bristles of the toothbrush are soft; remember, trauma to the gum tissue can lead to many of the manifestations you are trying to prevent. The head of the toothbrush should also be small enough to get to the hard-to-reach places in the back of the mouth. And remember, brush your tongue gently when brushing your teeth as well.

Floss Your Teeth Daily

Flossing is one thing that most people neglect, but, in fact, it is probably the best way to prevent tooth decay and dental problems. Flossing helps remove plaque that builds up between teeth in places brushing can't access. It also removes food particles that can help cause decay. Flossing has become easier with the advent of dental flossers—small disposable handles with floss at one end that makes flossing less cumbersome.

Regular Dental Exams and Cleanings

The one prevention means that can be pricey is regular dental exams and cleanings. If dental insurance is not available, the cost of seeing a dentist and hygienist can be steep. However, most commercial and government funded dental insurances do provide for these basic services at least once a year, some even twice each year. A dentist will examine not only your teeth for tooth decay, but your oral tissue as well. The dentist will look for any lesions, infections, or areas of inflammation that could signal that a serious HIV-related problem is brewing. The hygienist will do a very thorough cleaning of your teeth, much more thorough than you can do using a toothbrush and floss. Ideally, people should get a dental exam and cleaning at least every six months. However, people with a higher risk of oral disease should schedule these more than twice a year. Unfortunately, if insurance is an issue, this could be difficult. Talk with your HIV agency or case manager. Many states offer a dental assistance program for HIV patients who qualify. Many local communities have publically funded community dental clinics for those people without the means to pay for a private dentist.

Antimicrobial Mouth Rinses

Antimicrobial mouth rinses, such as Listerine©, can provide some additional prevention from the bacteria that can cause some of the most common oral conditions. However, using such a rinse does not replace the need to see a dentist regularly, and in many cases will not do much to prevent some of the more complex and serious manifestations of HIV.

KNOW YOUR MOUTH

We stress to anyone living with HIV to learn about their body and what is normal for you, so that when a change does occur you identify that change and can report the change to your physician. The same is true for your mouth. Examine your mouth on a regular basis. Keep an eye out for lesions, ulcerated areas, bleeding, loose teeth, etc., and report these things to your HIV specialist or dentist right away. If you develop pain (tooth pain, jaw pain, headaches, or tenderness of the oral tissue), report it to your physician and dentist as well. Early detection can be the difference between successful treatment and a long, hard road of dental and oral problems.

STOP SMOKING AND TOBACCO USE

Many people don't realize that smoking and tobacco use can be a major contributor to oral and dental disease. Tobacco use greatly increases your risk of oral cancers, gum disease, and tooth decay. Plus, smoking can slow down healing after oral procedures, and from oral diseases and infections. Stopping smoking is understandably one of the hardest things there is to do. Consult your HIV specialist or case manager, who can refer you to smoking cessation programs in your area.

Summary

Oral health and your overall health are more closely related than you may have originally thought. Clues to one's overall health can be gained by assessing the health of the mouth, teeth, and oral mucosa. In the HIV-positive person, oral health is extremely important, but, unfortunately, is an area that seems to have a low priority with patients and even some physicians. Literally all HIV patients will have some sort of oral manifestation sometime in the course of their infection. Therefore, it's very important to maintain the health of the mouth, teeth, and oral mucosa, just like it's important to maintain the health of the immune system. Make certain you see a dentist at least once a year, preferably twice each year; make certain you follow your dentist's advice and perform regular brushing and flossing; and finally, if you have any pain, lesions, loose teeth, or other abnormality in your mouth, notify your HIV physician right away. By maintaining good oral health, your overall health will be better as well.

13

Exercise and Nutrition

Nutrition

There's an old saying that goes "You are what you eat." In other words, your health and well being is largely dependent upon the types of food you eat. Eating lean meats, whole grains, and fish is a lot better for you than fast food, potato chips, and candy. The more nutritious the foods you eat the better you will feel. And in the case of people living with a chronic disease such as HIV, fighting that disease requires a higher number of calories, vitamins, and minerals. Unfortunately, as is the case with good dental care, people often place a lower priority on good nutrition. In actuality, good nutrition should be given the highest priority.

Studies show that nutritional status is a strong predictor of survival and functional status in people living with HIV. In other words, HIV-positive people who are struggling with poor nutrition will also struggle with their HIV. Nutritional interventions—those interventions that can improve nutrition—can have a very positive impact on mortality, morbidity, and the quality of life of those people living with HIV. For instance, nutritional counseling from a registered dietician has been proven to decrease hospitalizations and trips to the emergency room. Simply put, your body needs proper nutrition in order to heal and to maintain good health while living with HIV. Let's take a closer look at nutrition and diet and the role they play in the life of people living with HIV.

Barriers to Good Nutrition

Most everyone loves to eat, but eating just any old food isn't good enough. A healthy diet is one that has the right amount of fats, carbohydrates, proteins, and calories that meet a person's dietary needs. But when it comes to calories, more is less, meaning if you take in more calories than you need, the excess is stored as fats. Too much fat and you become overweight, a condition that can make treating any chronic disease, including HIV, much more difficult (not to mention the diseases that emerge as a result of being overweight, such as diabetes and heart disease, to name just two). Along with the proper number and types of vitamins and minerals, a proper diet can significantly enhance your health and ability to fight your HIV. But, unfortunately, many people find there are barriers to eating right — barriers that interfere with a proper diet. Let's look at some of those barriers.

POOR HEALTH AND NOT FEELING WELL

If you are living with HIV, the reality is that there are times you just don't feel well. Nausea caused by opportunistic infections, HIV medications, or by HIV itself makes it very difficult to eat a proper diet. Vomiting, abdominal pain, or diarrhea can leave you with little or no appetite, making it difficult to eat a nutritious meal, which in turn makes it unlikely you will get the calories and nutrients you require. Losing your appetite can happen on occasion, and it typically will return in a couple of days. Keep in mind that as long as you are drinking the proper amount and type of fluids each day, a decreased appetite for a short period of time is nothing to worry about. However, if your appetite doesn't improve after three to four days, or you are losing weight as a result of not eating, you should contact your doctor.

While poor health can make it difficult to eat a nutritious meal, the symptoms that accompany your HIV can make it difficult to prepare one as well. Standing at your kitchen counter to prepare your breakfast, lunch, or dinner can be made difficult by the fatigue and weakness that sometimes accompanies HIV. Nausea and vomiting can make handling or smelling foods undesirable. Typically, nutritious meals do require more preparation than do those foods offering little in the way of nutrients. Meals that require minimal preparation time and effort are usually those with the least amount of nutrients. In most cases this means processed foods such as "TV dinners," boxed meals, or the worst case scenario—fast food. While these foods provide calories, they offer little else in the way of nutrients. In fact, these types of food provide excessive amounts of fat, sugars, salt, and artificial ingredients that do little to improve the nutritional status of the HIV-positive person.

ORAL LESIONS, MOUTH PAIN, OR TOOTH PAIN

As we discussed in previous chapters of this book, oral manifestations of HIV are common occurrences for most people living with HIV. Oral lesions, ulcers, mouth pain or infections common to HIV can interfere with eating and drinking, and, in turn, with proper nutrition. Poor dental hygiene will eventually cause tooth decay and painful dental caries (cavities), making it difficult to eat. Viral infections such as herpes; fungal infections such as thrush (candidiasis or yeast); and bacterial infections such as periodontitis (infection of the gum tissue) cause mild to severe pain that makes eating difficult to impossible, sometimes affecting appetite as well. If you can't eat, you can't maintain proper nutrition. Therefore, maintaining optimal dental health is essential to good nutrition.

FINANCIAL RESOURCES

When money is tight, people find ways to cut costs and save a few dollars. Preparing healthy meals at home can be too expensive for someone on a fixed income or who has limited financial resources. Unfortunately, fast food is not a good source of nutrition. But for people with a limited income, foods high in nutrients may be too expensive for their budget. Luckily, there are publically-funded programs, such as the food stamp program, that help people buy nutritious food and thereby decrease the amount of fast food in their diet. Many HIV treatment programs employ dieticians that can assist low income families in planning nutritious meals using foods that fit into a limited budget. There are local community agencies that sponsor food banks that collect donations of food and money from the community and make it available to those people in need. However, because they rely on donations, the availability of these resources is limited. Supplies are rationed to insure as many people as possible get something, meaning what they receive may not go far in terms of feeding a family.

BEING HOMELESS

For those people who are homeless, buying and storing food is impossible. There are homeless shelters and soup kitchens that try to provide nutritious meals, but, like with food banks, funding is very limited, and shelters most often rely on donations and volunteers to acquire and prepare the food. Because of limited supplies and the number of homeless people they need to feed, agencies may limit individuals to one meal each day, or, in extreme circumstances, only offer meals on holidays like Christmas and Thanksgiving. In addition to the limited availability of food, there is a relatively high incidence of alcoholism and drug use among the homeless. In these individuals, if resources are available they are typically used to buy alcohol or drugs, foregoing nutrition in order to satisfy their addiction.

POOR MOBILITY OR TRANSPORTATION

Depending on the overall health and the living situation of the individual, acquiring food can be a challenge. If their medical status impedes their mobility, or they are without reliable transportation, getting to the grocery store to purchase food is difficult. Being confined to their home, they must rely on others to bring them the food they need. For those whose mobility is limited, preparing meals may be difficult, as we discussed earlier in this chapter. In some large urban areas there are agencies that provide volunteers who shop and deliver groceries for those who are unable to do so for themselves. Some grocery stores or private businesses offer food shopping and delivery for a fee. Ideally, a neighbor, a loved one, or a family member is available to help out.

The Nutritional Impact of HIV

We know that HIV impacts every aspect of your health and body. The HIV program I work in has a slogan that goes something like this: "Because we realize HIV impacts your life in so many ways."

And certainly nutritional status is one of those ways. We've shown that diet and nutrition can have a great deal of impact on your health and how well you live with HIV. To illustrate this point further, HIV's impact on nutrition is classified into three categories.

INADEQUATE INTAKE

In any disease state, including HIV, the human body needs increased amounts of calories and nutrients to fight their disease and to heal completely. One would think by just eating, your body's nutrient requirements would be met. But HIV and conditions associated with the virus makes that easier said than done. HIV increases the body's metabolic needs, meaning nutrients such as protein and carbohydrates are being used at an accelerated rate. The body's energy requirements are also increased, meaning the number of calories the body needs to produce that energy increases as well. But keep in mind that not just any calories will do. The body needs calories that are made up of nutrients that satisfy the body's many nutritional needs during this increased metabolic state. For instance, you can increase your calories by eating either potato chips or baked fish, but it's the baked fish that will offer you the best kind of calories—those complete with the proper nutrients, vitamins, and minerals that are required for the body to fight your disease. Potato chips and foods like them provide what are called "empty calories"—those calories that offer very little in terms of nutrients.

There are many causes for inadequate intake of nutrients in the HIV-positive person. The most common cause is nausea and vomiting, most often a side effect of HIV medications. Altered taste and poor appetite can also affect nutrient intake and can be a medication side effect as well. Associated illnesses, like HIV wasting or opportunistic infections, specifically those of the gastrointestinal (GI) tract, also make it very difficult to take in the nutrients essential to a healthy life.

Poor Absorption of Nutrients

You can take in all the nutrients you want, but without the proper absorption of those nutrients they'll do you no good at all. In the absence of HIV, opportunistic infections, or other disease states, absorption is a natural process of utilizing the food we eat by absorbing the nutrients contained in that food. However, in the presence of HIV, absorption is often compromised, most often caused by infections of the GI tract or damage to the GI tract by HIV itself. Normally, nutrients are absorbed through the walls of the intestines. But infections or damage to the absorptive surfaces of the gastric mucosa interferes with the normal absorption of nutrients, vitamins, and minerals. Diarrhea and increased gastric motility (movement) through the intestinal tract can also interfere with the body's ability to absorb nutrients. For absorption to occur, the digesting food and gastric acid mixture must have contact with the walls of the intestinal tract. But if that mixture is moving too fast through the GI tract, there is not enough time for proper absorption to occur, and most of the nutrients are lost in the form of diarrhea.

Altered Metabolism of Nutrients

Metabolism is defined as the sum total of all the chemical and physical processes occurring in a living organism. It's the metabolic process that uses food and oxygen we take in to produce the energy and basic materials needed for life processes. In a healthy body, metabolism is a finely tuned process of converting what we take in each day into the energy, proteins, fats and carbohydrates we need for life processes. Metabolism is also responsible for the breakdown and excretion of waste products, medications, and harmful substances that may enter the body. HIV can alter metabolism and the way in which our bodies process, utilize, store, and excrete the nutrients we take in each day. Other factors, including immune system dysfunction, medication side effects, opportunistic infections, and hormonal changes, can also alter metabolism. Conditions commonly associated with HIV, including poorly controlled blood sugar, lipodystrophy, and elevated cholesterol and triglyceride levels, are all evidence of the disruptive effects HIV can have on metabolism.

What Is a Good Diet?

When watching television or reading the newspaper, terms such as "*proper nutrition*" and "*a good diet*" pop up over and over. But what exactly do those terms mean? What constitutes a good diet? What is meant by proper nutrition? A simple definition of proper nutrition or a good diet could go something like: "*a diet that provides all the daily required vitamins and minerals with the right balance of calories, fats, carbohydrates (sugars), and protein.*" Pardon the pun, but that's a mouthful. Luckily, there are established standards and guidelines for what we are calling a good diet. Let's look at the different aspects of a good diet and proper nutrition.

CALORIES

The scientific definition of a calorie is *the amount of heat needed to raise the temperature of one gram of water one degree celsius.* But that definition really does little for you when trying to put together a healthy diet. A better definition may be that a calorie measures *the amount of energy contained in the foods we eat.* For instance, the six ounce steak you eat provides energy in the form of calories, fueling the body's processes. In other words, calories are the fuel that powers our body. So where do we find these calories? As we've already mentioned, calories are found in three different forms and are contained in the foods we eat. Let's examine those three forms.

Carbohydrates

Carbohydrates (sugars) are the body's primary source of energy, providing four calories for every gram of carbohydrates. Depending on the size of the molecule, they can be complex or simple. The small-molecule carbohydrates are in the form of simple sugars—namely, glucose and fructose. Honey, fresh fruit, and dairy products contain these simple sugars. Because of their small molecular size, they can be broken down for energy very quickly. However, their energy lasts only a short time. Under certain circumstances, simple sugars can chain together and form large, complex sugars. These sugars can also be broken down for energy relatively quickly but last longer than do the simple sugars. Examples of complex carbohydrates include breads, grains, vegetables, and pasta.

Fats

These complex molecules are comprised of substances called *fatty acids.* When energy is needed and there is a shortage of carbohydrates (sugars), fats are broken down into fatty acids, and they, in turn, are burned for energy. Fats are a major source of energy for the body, released slowly but efficiently. Because they are such an efficient source of energy, the body stores its excess calories as fat beneath the skin (subcutaneous), in certain organs such as the liver, and within the walls of blood vessels. There are nine calories stored in every gram of fat. This is more than twice the amount of calories as the same amount of proteins or carbohydrates. Because there are certain fatty acids the body can't manufacture, fats must be taken in as part of a healthy diet. However, fat need only be taken in to a certain extent. Excessive fats in the diet get deposited throughout the body and contribute to such health conditions as obesity, high blood pressure, diabetes, and heart and vascular disease.

Proteins

Proteins are comprised of molecules called amino acids, strung together to form large, complex molecules. Because they are so large, the energy in protein is released slowly and lasts longer than carbohydrates (sugars) or fats. Proteins are the building blocks of the human body, providing substances needed to manufacture skin, muscles, and bone. For every gram of protein in the diet, four calories of energy is available for use by the body. While most amino acids are produced in the body, some need to be taken in as part of the diet. Any protein not immediately used is broken down by the body, and its component parts are stored as fat.

VITAMINS

Another part of a good diet and proper nutrition are vitamins. A vitamin is a small molecule that your body needs in minute quantities in order to carry out body processes and chemical reactions. Vitamins act as catalysts—those compounds that "kick start" or initiate chemical reactions in the body. Like the match that starts the fire, vitamins start chemical reactions and, in some cases, speed up reactions necessary for life. Vitamins are either fat soluble or water soluble, meaning they either dissolve in water or in fat. But vitamins aren't manufactured by the body, so they must be taken in with the foods we eat, or they must be taken as supplements (for example, once-a-day vitamins). There are thirteen different vitamins that are considered essential to a healthy life. These vitamins are absolutely necessary if the body is to function properly. Let's look at some of these essential vitamins.

Vitamin A

Vitamin A is a fat soluble vitamin also known as Retinol. This essential vitamin is produced in the stomach by the enzymatic breakdown of beta-carotene, a naturally occurring nutrient found in plants and vegetables. The vitamin A produced in the stomach in turn produces the substance retinal, which is used by the rods and cones of the eye to sense light. It's this fact that has spawned the belief that eating carrots (a source of beta-carotene) is good for your eyes. In fact, this is more accurate than you may think. Your body can't make retinal without Vitamin A, and you can't see without retinal; therefore, sources of vitamin A, such as carrots are good for your eyesight. It being a fat soluble vitamin, it is possible to take in too much vitamin A. Typically, this is a result of taking excessive amounts of vitamin supplements.

Vitamin B

The B vitamins are actually a collection of eight water soluble vitamins that are referred to as the *B complex vitamins*. The B complex vitamins perform many functions, including breaking down carbohydrates for energy;

breaking down proteins and fats for the normal functioning of the nervous system; and maintaining normal muscle tone in the stomach and intestinal tract. The B complex vitamins include:

- B1—thiamine
- B2—riboflavin
- B3—niacin
- B5—pantothenic acid
- B6—pyridoxine
- B12—cyanocobalamin
- folic acid
- biotin

Vitamin C

Also known as ascorbic acid, vitamin C is the most well know but least understood of all the vitamins. A very important vitamin, it's responsible for the production of collagen, which is needed for healthy bones, teeth, gums and blood vessels; it acts as a strong antioxidant (substances that protect other tissues, cells membranes, and other vitamins from the damaging effects of oxygen); it controls and helps limit infections; and it treats diseases such as anemia and scurvy (vitamin C deficiency). There has been some conjecture that large daily doses of vitamin C will prevent the common cold. Unfortunately, that theory has not panned out. Studies have shown that while the doses of vitamin C found in a once-a-day vitamin may ease the symptoms of a cold, there is no proof that once-a-day dosage or higher doses will prevent a cold from occurring.

Vitamin D

The only vitamin produced by the body, this fat soluble vitamin is important in the absorption and retention of calcium and phosphorous, both essential minerals found in healthy bones and teeth. Very few foods have significant quantities of vitamin D. Milk and breakfast cereals, both fortified with vitamin D in the manufacturing process, are the best dietary sources of the vitamin. Some fish are also good sources of vitamin D. While few dietary sources of vitamin D exist, it is produced naturally by the body. When the sunlight's ultraviolet rays strike the skin, a photochemical reaction occurs, producing vitamin D. Technically, vitamin D is considered a hormone because of its regulatory role in the absorption and excretion of calcium. There is also evidence that vitamin D strengthens the immune system and even prevents some types of cancer. As was mentioned earlier, few foods provide vitamin D unless the food has been vitamin enriched during the manufacturing process. Therefore, in order to get the daily required amounts of vitamin D, a once-a-day multivitamin is recommended.

Vitamin E

As one of the fat soluble vitamins, vitamin E acts as a powerful antioxidant that protects cell membranes from the damage caused by oxidation. The vitamin also increases the availability of vitamin A by inhibiting its intestinal oxidation. When vitamin A is in the intestinal tract, its structure is changed and destroyed by coming in contact with oxygen molecules (oxidation). Vitamin E inhibits this process, making more vitamin A available for body processes. Vitamin E is found in foods derived from plants, such as wheat germ and whole grains. Other foods, such as nuts, peanut butter, and vegetable oils, are also good sources of vitamin E. Early studies suggested that vitamin E may help decrease the risk of cardiac disease by slowing the oxidation of bad cholesterol (LDL), which produces the fatty plaques that contribute to arterial narrowing and the formation of blood clots that eventually lead to heart attacks. However, there is some recent evidence that caution is warranted when suggesting vitamin E in those cardiac patients taking drugs to lower their cholesterol. The combination of the two has been known to inhibit the anti-inflammatory action of cholesterol-lowering drugs, which actually increases the risk of heart disease in those patients. Experts continue to suggest vitamin E be taken by those patients not taking cholesterol-lowering drugs, keeping in mind, however, that in order for vitamin E to have arterial benefits (benefits to your blood vessels), it must be taken along with vitamin C.

Vitamin K

Another of the fat soluble vitamins, vitamin K is necessary for normal blood clotting and the production of proteins needed for plasma, bone and kidney production. In addition, its antioxidant properties protect the skin from the negative effects of oxidation. The primary sources of vitamin K are leafy green vegetables, such as kale, cabbage, and broccoli, which together provide about half of the dietary requirement. The remainder of necessary vitamin K comes from such things as wheat bran, cereals, certain fruits, dairy products, and eggs. While healthy adults typically have plenty of vitamin K, infants and especially newborns commonly have deficiencies. In fact, vitamin K is routinely given to newborns to protect against blood clotting difficulties that occur with vitamin K deficiencies.

MINERALS

As important as vitamins are to a healthy body, they can do very little without the catalytic actions of minerals. Like vitamins, minerals are substances needed in very small amounts in order for the body to function properly. Outside of the body or by themselves, minerals do very little. But in the body they function as catalysts, meaning they help initiate biological reactions—reactions that are necessary for life. Examples of these reactions include such processes as transmission of nervous impulses, proper muscle function, and the utilization of nutrients in the foods we eat.

Many people equate vitamins and minerals, but in actuality they are really quite different. While the two do function together, there is one very important difference. Vitamins are organic, meaning they contain carbon atoms. Minerals, on the other hand, are inorganic, meaning they contain no carbon atoms. There are some vitamins that can be produced in the body. However, the absence of carbon atoms means the body is unable to produce minerals naturally. Instead, essential minerals come from a healthy diet and dietary supplements, such as once-a-day multivitamins. There are hundreds of minerals found in the body, but twenty-five are considered essential to a healthy life. These twenty-five minerals are divided into two main categories:

Macrominerals

These minerals are required by the body in amounts greater than or equal to 100mg per day. Some examples of macrominerals include calcium, magnesium, sodium, potassium, phosphorus and chlorine. These minerals are found in virtually every cell in the body and are essential to bodily functions, such as muscle contraction, heart function, and bone growth. Granted, dietary causes of mineral deficiency are rare, but keep in mind that insufficient quantities of certain minerals, such as potassium, can cause severe illness or even death.

Microminerals

Also known as trace minerals or micronutrients, these are chemical elements needed by the body in quantities less than 100mg per day. Examples include elements such as iron, cobalt, chromium, copper, iodine, manganese, selenium, zinc, and molybdenum. Despite being used in such minute quantities, trace minerals perform many important roles and functions. Trace minerals are necessary for oxygen transport throughout the body; the uptake of nutrients, including vitamins and other minerals; proper hormone and enzyme function; and, finally, the breakdown of nutrients to produce energy.

A Word About Oxidation

When most people think about oxidation, the first thing that comes to mind is the rust that forms on the fenders of an old car. Years of moisture on exposed metal causes a layer of rust to form. If left untreated, rust can eat its way through a car's bumper or door in no time. But oxidation is not limited to the body of a car. In fact, oxidation can do great harm to the human body as well. Technically speaking, oxidation is the process by which substances interact with oxygen, causing that substance to lose electrons. Those lost electrons cause the release of reactive substances known as free radicals. Circulating free radicals stress and damage cells throughout the body. The natural aging process is an example of the damaging effects of free radicals and oxidation.

Obviously, we are all going to age over time. However, certain foods, vitamins, and minerals act as antioxidants, slowing the damage done by oxidation. For instance, certain compounds found in dark chocolate and red wine are known to have antioxidant properties. Many antioxidants are often identified in food by their distinctive colors. For example, the deep red of cherries and tomatoes; the orange of carrots; the yellow of corn, mangos, and saffron; and the blue-purple of blueberries, blackberries, and grapes are all examples of antioxidants. Finally, vitamin E has long been considered to be a vitamin that can ward off the aging process. Obviously, we will all age, despite vitamin E and other antioxidants. But the inclusion of antioxidants in our diet can help our bodies stay healthier longer.

How Much of These Nutrients Do We Need?

Now that we know what is included in a healthy diet, it's important for us to know how much of these things we need in order to stay healthy. You have probably heard the old adage *"too much of a good thing."* That goes for nutrition as well. You need plenty of calories, fats, proteins, vitamins and minerals to stay healthy. However, too much of any of these things and your health can be compromised.

Vitamins, Minerals, and HIV

Vitamins and minerals are referred to as micronutrients because the body requires them in very small amounts to function properly. Studies indicate that people living with HIV have a greater risk of developing micronutrient deficiencies. And, in fact, the recommended daily requirements of micronutrients are greater in people living with HIV compared to those who are HIV-negative. Furthermore, deficiencies in required nutrients will increase the probability that HIV will progress to AIDS. Because of the increased risk inherent to HIV-infected people, experts agree that people living with HIV should take a multivitamin, complete with essential minerals, once each day to reduce the risk of micronutrient deficiencies.

The Role of Antioxidants in HIV

Earlier in this chapter we discussed oxidation and the role antioxidants play in staying healthy. As a review, antioxidants are vitamins, minerals, and other nutrients found in foods or produced by the body that protect cells from circulating reactive substances called free radicals. Free radicals are released as a result of oxidation, the interaction of oxygen and substances within the body. Circulating free radicals can stress and damage cells throughout the body.

Typically, the body maintains a balance between free radicals and antioxidants that take care of them. But chronic infections, such as HIV, can throw that balance off, meaning there are greater numbers of free radicals—too many, in fact, for the body to handle. Exposure to such things as toxic chemicals or cigarette smoke can also add to the number of circulating free radicals. This free radical imbalance is sometimes referred to as *oxidative stress*—in other words, stress placed on the cells of the body due to increased numbers of circulating free radicals. Boosting the body's antioxidants will help handle the oxidative stress and slow the damaging effects of oxidation. Certain vitamins and minerals act as antioxidants, boosting the body's natural defenses against the deleterious effects of free radicals and oxidative stress.

Get Help with Your Nutrition

For those people living with HIV, there are so many issues that need attention. Medications need to be taken on time each and every day. Regular visits to your HIV specialist need to be scheduled and kept. There are issues with your employer, your finances, and your relationships. There are times you will feel sad; times you will feel happy; times you will feel alone; and times you will feel anxious. Finally, there are concerns of prejudice, stereotypes, and mistreatment. With so much on your mind, and additional stresses being added all the time, how in the world can you understand the complexities of nutrition and put together a healthy diet, too? The fact is you are going to need help and guidance to get your diet and nutritional state into the best shape it can be. You are going to need a dietician.

The Role of the Dietician

The management of HIV is a very complex and difficult task for provider and patient alike. With the advent of new medications and treatments, people are living longer and, as a result, need expertise in all areas of HIV care over the course of their lives. With the emergence of metabolic problems such as elevated cholesterol and triglycerides, lipodystrophy, and blood sugar dysfunction, nutritional expertise is needed now more than ever. A registered dietician can provide that expertise.

Experts agree that it has become evident over the course of the epidemic that all people living with HIV should have access to a registered dietician—

ideally, one with expertise in HIV and AIDS as well as nutrition. In fact, nutrition and proper diet are so important to the HIV-positive person that experts recommend that HIV care programs employ a registered dietician or have a dietician available for referral — again, one with an expertise in HIV and AIDS. The roles of the dietician would include such things as nutrition screenings, counseling, education, and medical referral, to name just a few. Let's take a closer look at ways a dietician can help people living with HIV and AIDS.

Screening / Referral / Assessment

Obviously, before any nutritional issues can be addressed they have to be identified. A thorough nutrition screening is necessary to identify any problems or deficiencies. The screening should include a complete medical and nutrition history; body measurements that include *body fat composition* (percentage of total body weight that is fat) and *body mass index* (BMI — a comparison of body weight to height); and a complete set of blood tests, including cholesterol and triglyceride levels, electrolytes, blood counts, and kidney and liver function. Keep in mind that a nutrition screening should be done as soon as possible after entrance into HIV care, and any time that the clinical picture suggests that there is a nutrition problem. Depending on the nutritional needs and risks of the HIV-positive person, the American Dietetic Association classifies nutrition risk in one of three categories.

- *High Risk*—people with two or more medical conditions or those having a weight loss of greater than 10 percent of their body weight over four to six months should ideally be seen by a dietician within one week of their entrance into HIV care.
- *Moderate Risk*—people suffering from chronic conditions such as chronic nausea, vomiting, and diarrhea, or those having signs of lipodystrophy, should been seen no later than one month after entry into HIV care.
- *Low Risk*—people without signs or symptoms of poor nutrition should be seen by a dietician at least once for an initial screening, and then again only as needed.

Once an issue has been identified, the patient should have a complete examination to assess how the identified nutritional issue is affecting overall health. This exam should include an evaluation of physical appearance and function. Does the patient look thin; is the skin dry and cracked; is there weakness or muscle atrophy; is the patient overweight or underweight when compared to height and body type; how much of the body's composition is fat; and finally, what is the waist and abdominal girth? All these factors are important in assessing the nutritional status of the HIV-positive person.

One other area that must be evaluated is the need for special dietary considerations. Are there issues that may affect the person's ability to eat, such has poor dental health, mouth pain, jaw pain, or absence of teeth altogether? Other considerations include such questions as what are the person's eating habits; what foods does the person like or dislike; is there any alteration in taste or smell that may interfere with eating; is the person taking vitamins or supplements; and finally, are there cultural requirements, financial factors, or problems with living arrangements (i.e. homelessness) that may affect nutrition or the ability to take in nutrients.

Treatment and Interventions

The key to avoiding nutritional deficiencies in the HIV positive person is initiating nutritional interventions soon after the diagnosis of HIV is made. Early access to nutritional care can help prevent malnutrition, lipodystrophy, and AIDS wasting syndrome. Preventing problems with nutrition starts with education. One of the primary roles of the dietician is to provide basic nutritional education to the HIV-positive patient, thereby providing that person with the tools to improve their nutritional status. Nutrition awareness and education allows people to identify problems early and take steps to avoid and correct problems in their diet.

Besides education, the dietician can refer patients to medical providers in order to treat the underlying cause of any nutritional deficiencies that may be present. For instance, if there is pain from an infected tooth preventing a patient from eating, the dietician can refer the person to a dentist who will treat the infection, making it possible for the patient to eat again. If there are financial issues preventing the patient from getting enough food, a referral to case management or social services can be made to help the patient obtain food via food banks, mobile meals programs, or food stamp programs. A medical referral can be made to evaluate and treat the cause or causes of diarrhea, vomiting, or other medical problems that may be interfering with proper nutrition.

Finally, metabolic problems such as elevated cholesterol and triglycerides, elevated blood sugar, aids wasting, and lipodystrophy can all be addressed through medical referral by the dietician.

Nutritional Counseling

Countless studies have proven that nutrition counseling from a registered dietician greatly improves outcomes and facilitates adequate nutritional intake for those people living with HIV. Nutrition counseling can provide the patient with methods that will help overcome barriers to good nutrition. These methods can be explored in a cooperative effort between the dietician and the person living with HIV. Part of nutritional counseling and education may include topics such as alternative therapies, naturopathic treatments, holistic medicine, and "fad" diets. A dietician can also teach you how to read the food nutrition label that is on everything you buy at the grocery story. Understanding these labels can help you choose food that is perfect for your needs. Making the HIV-positive person aware of the pros and cons of their diet can insure that patients have the tools necessary to make informed decisions regarding their nutritional status.

The importance of good nutrition and timely nutritional interventions can't be overstated. Proper nutrition, adequate nutrient intake, and the elimination of nutritional deficiencies are essential to a healthy life with HIV.

Much of what we must do to stay healthy involves choices. People choose to start smoking or choose to have that second bowl of ice cream. Making the right choices can mean the difference between being sick and being healthy. The importance of one such choice is often underestimated — the choice to exercise each day. We all know its importance, but all of us have come up with reasons why today is not a good day to start exercising. For people living with a chronic illness, regular exercise is especially important. Exercising even twenty minutes every other day can improve your body's ability to fight infection, can improve heart function, and can help maintain an optimal body weight. Let's take a look at exercise and how it plays a role in living healthy with HIV.

The Role of Exercise in HIV

It's no secret; whether you have HIV, diabetes, asthma, or don't have a chronic illness at all, exercise is beneficial to your overall health. In fact, you really can't be your healthiest without having exercise as part of your life. Keeping your body in tip-top shape can only be accomplished if you are physically active. The human body is like no other machine. A car will eventually breakdown with daily use: its tires wear down; the breaks wear down; even the paint fades and becomes scratched. If you want your car to last longer, put it in the garage and drive the car very little. The human body, unlike your car, will break down with inactivity. If you lay in bed for a few days, you will become weak, stiff, and very fatigued. Unlike other machines, the human body needs to be active in order to stay healthy. Without exercise, your body will break down, and you will not be as healthy as you could be. While these facts are true for each one of us, exercise is especially beneficial for people living with chronic illnesses such as HIV. There are several advantages and benefits to regular exercise. Here are just a few:

- Improved muscle mass, strength, and endurance.
- Improved heart and lung function and endurance.
- Increased energy levels throughout the day.
- Reduced stress and enhanced sense of well being.
- Strengthened immune system, including boosted CD4 counts in some people.

- Increased bone strength.
- Decreased cholesterol and triglycerides.
- Better controlled weight gain and decreased fat accumulation.
- Improved metabolism and the way the body uses and controls blood sugar.
- Improved sleep.

So, given its benefits, it's obvious we should include a program of regular exercise in our daily lives. However, there can be risks when starting an exercise program. Everybody can benefit from some degree of regular exercise — as long as the exercise program is geared to the person's physical abilities and takes into account their physical and emotional limitations. For instance, running ten miles each day will benefit a professional athlete, but it would probably do great harm to a 75-year-old grandmother. Lifting weights each day is a good way to build strength unless you are recovering from a dislocated shoulder. Exercise programs must take into consideration past injuries, health problems, current physical condition, and current medical conditions in order to be beneficial. Here are some factors to consider before starting any exercise program.

- Exercising beyond your abilities or limitations can actually be harmful. Before starting any exercise program, have a complete physical exam by your physician. Ask for specific recommendations regarding the level of exercise that is right for you. If you have access to a dietician or personal trainer, ask for their recommendations as well. Start slow, building strength and endurance before moving to the next level of exercise. For instance, start by running a half mile each day, moving to one mile each day only after being able to run the half mile comfortably. When weightlifting, start at lighter weights and move up as you get stronger.
- Because body fluid loss increases during rigorous exercise, the amount of fluids taken in must be increased to avoid dehydration. Dehydration can be a very serious condition, especially in the elderly, in children, and in people with chronic illnesses such as HIV. Keep in mind that fluid replacement should be in the form of water or electrolyte replacement drinks like Pedialyte or Gatorade. Caffeinated beverages like soda or tea actually makes dehydration worse and should be avoided.
- Regular exercise will cause weight loss. Excess body fat will be the first to go, but people who have very little body fat will lose lean body mass (muscle) instead. If you are overweight, losing excess fat will make you healthier. If, like many HIV-positive people, you have very little body fat, losing lean body mass can be a problem. Therefore, if you choose to exercise and wish to maintain your lean body mass, you must increase your caloric intake to match the increased caloric requirements of exercise. In addition, a diet with the proper amounts of fats, carbohydrates, and proteins must take into consideration the increased needs caused by exercising.

- As careful as we are or try to be, exercise can lead to injuries. To avoid injuries during your exercise, make certain you are performing the exercises correctly. For instance, if you are lifting weights, make sure you are using proper body mechanics to avoid pulled muscles, torn tendons, and muscle strains and sprains. If your exercise regimen employs exercise equipment, learn how to operate the equipment properly and safely before starting your exercise program. Heard of the phrase *"No pain no gain"*? Ignore that phrase and not the pain you are having. Pain is a sign that injury has occurred or may occur if exercise continues. Ignoring the signs of pain can cause or worsen injuries. If you do sustain an injury, see your doctor and suspend your exercise program until your injury is completely healed.

- Give your body a chance to recover. During exercise, muscles experience stress and some degree of trauma. By exercising only every other day, your muscles are given a chance to recover from the stress of exercise. If you prefer to exercise every day, change the type of exercise you do every other day. For instance, do aerobic exercises (i.e. running) on odd numbered days and weight training on even numbered days. Make sure you incorporate one day of rest each week in order to allow your body to fully recover.

Exercise Tips and Suggestions

Once you obtain medical clearance from your doctor and you understand how to exercise safely, you can begin your exercise program. But before you begin, take a look at these tips and suggestions that will make your exercise program safer and much more beneficial.

Know Your Limitations

Just because exercise is good for you doesn't mean more exercise is better. In fact, too much exercise, or exercising more than your body is able to tolerate, can be harmful. Remember the old adage "Everything in moderation." The same holds true for exercise. Start slowly, three times per week, for instance, allowing your body to build up strength and endurance. As your strength and endurance improve, increase the amount of exercise and the difficulty of the exercises you are doing. Even this smallest amount of exercise will have an impact on your overall health. You will build muscle, lose excess weight, and feel better in the process. Keep in mind that your progress may be slow or you may find it hard to exercise due to fatigue or other medical issues. Take it slow, be patient, and do only what your body allows. Remember, any exercise is better than none.

Proper Diet Is Key

As we discussed earlier in this chapter, proper diet and nutrition is an important part of staying healthy. If you exercise regularly, a proper diet is especially important. Keep in mind your diet must be adjusted according to the goal of your exercise program. If you are trying to lose weight and burn excess fat, then decreasing your calorie and fat intake is necessary. However, if you are trying to build muscle and lean body mass, then a diet with increased calories and protein is necessary. Keep in mind that if you do not want to lose or gain weight, then your calorie intake must be about the same as the amount burned while exercising.

Keep in mind that not just any calories will do. The calories you take in must be "good calories"—calories that are part of a nutritious diet. For instance, a person can increase their calorie intake by eating nothing but potato chips every day. However, those types of calories are nothing but "empty calories," meaning they are calories that will do nothing but add to your fat stores. Instead, a person would be better served by increasing their calories by eating fish or lean meats, foods that will help build lean body mass.

Drink Plenty of Fluids to Avoid Dehydration

Another important aspect of any exercise program is proper fluid intake. During exercise, your body loses large quantities of bodily fluids due to perspiration and body temperature regulation. Exercise generates body heat that must be dissipated in order to maintain proper body temperature. Body temperature is largely regulated by perspiring. Exertion causes sweat or perspiration to form on the surface of the skin. As the sweat evaporates, it takes excess heat away from the body, and in doing so restores the body's normal temperature. It's hard to believe that the amount of water lost through sweating is enough to cause dehydration. But it certainly is, and therefore must be replaced by drinking the proper amount and type of fluid. If fluid is not replaced, the bloodstream and cells throughout the body become fluid depleted. In addition, fluid depletion also causes electrolyte (mineral) imbalances. These imbalances can affect muscle, nerve and heart function. It's obvious that during exercise it is extremely important to replace bodily fluids in order to avoid dehydration.

Learn to recognize the signs and symptoms of dehydration, and what to do if you do become dehydrated. Symptoms include:

- dry skin, tongue, or other mucous membranes;
- fever;
- headache, lightheadedness, or dizziness, especially when changing position;
- low blood pressure and high heart rate.

Mild dehydration may be nothing more than an uncomfortable inconvenience. If left untreated, however, it can become a serious, potentially fatal condition. So when you feel the signs and symptoms of dehydration coming on, it's important not to ignore them. Fluid replacement is of utmost importance, but treating dehydration is more than just drinking water. Granted, drinking water will replace the fluids you have lost, but there is still the matter of electrolyte imbalances common in dehydration. Electrolyte solutions such as Pedialyte or Gatorade can be used to replace both fluids and electrolytes. Eating fresh fruits such as oranges and bananas, or drinking soup broth that contains sodium (salt) is also a good way to replenish the minerals lost during exercise. Be careful to avoid energy drinks, soda, or other caffeinated beverages. Caffeine can actually make dehydration worse.

The best way to treat dehydration is to avoid it altogether. Water or electrolyte solutions should be taken during and after exercise or physical exertion to keep up with fluids lost through perspiration. Avoiding dehydration will make exercise less difficult and will help you avoid potential problems afterward.

Enjoy Your Exercise Program

I'll be the first to admit that as much as I tout the benefits of exercise, it's not always fun and entertaining. In fact, exercise can be downright unpleasant. It's the unpleasantness that makes it so hard to continue your exercise program. So it makes sense to choose a type of exercise or a program of exercise that you will enjoy. For instance, it makes little sense to include jogging in your exercise program if you hate to jog. If you don't care for weightlifting, choose another means of building and toning muscle. If you like what you're doing it will be much easier to stick to your regimen. If you like rollerblading, add that to your exercise program. If swimming is more your cup of tea, jump in feet first (pardon the pun). You have to like what you're doing in order to stick with the program.

Another reason why people can't seem to stick to their exercise program is boredom. People get tired of doing the same thing day in and day out, regardless of how much they typically enjoy the activity. You may love to rollerblade, but if you have to do that an hour each day every day as part of your regular exercise program you can count on becoming bored eventually. Variety is the spice of life it is said. The same holds true for exercise. If you get bored, you will find it harder to stick to the program. If you find it's becoming harder to find the ambition and motivation to exercise, try changing up your routine a bit. Instead of rollerblading on Wednesdays, ride your bike. If you're tired of jogging every other day, join an aerobics class instead. Boredom can destroy your motivation no matter how intent you are on getting healthier. Motivation is the key to any exercise program, and variety will keep you motivated while making exercise more fun.

Summary

Done properly and within the limitations of your body and your health, exercise will increase strength, reduce stress levels, improve the health of your immune system, help control cholesterol and triglyceride levels, maintain an optimal body weight, and improve metabolism, endurance and cardiac health. Exercise in some form should be a part of everyone's day, even as little as thirty minutes every other day. But remember, before starting any program of exercise, consult your doctor. He or she can help you design a program of exercise that will be right for you.

14

Living with HIV

It's time to bring it all together. For thirteen chapters we discussed everything from HIV prevention to HIV diagnosis and beyond. We have talked about
medications, opportunistic infections, exercise and nutrition. But the purpose
of this text is to make living with HIV easier. Day to day life with HIV can be
a challenge, but hopefully this text will make that challenge less imposing. Our
last chapter is called "Living with HIV," and that's exactly what we are going
to discuss. This last chapter offers information that will help you handle the
practical side of HIV, those issues most everyone faces but that are made more
difficult because of an HIV diagnosis. The first topic we will cover is the special concerns of women living with HIV.

The Special Needs of Women Living with HIV

Like all chronic diseases, HIV can make life more complicated at times.
No longer considered a terminal illness, HIV will, however, change your life.
Experts agree that while HIV will impact the lives of all who are infected, women
have a unique set of issues that must be dealt with. From opportunistic infections to social issues, the impact of HIV on the life of a woman is very different than its impact on a man. For example, everyone living with HIV must
understand and be concerned with medications, opportunistic infections, and
safer sex. But women have those concerns and more. For instance, an HIV-positive woman of child bearing age has to be aware of the risks some HIV medicines pose if she were to get pregnant. Her male counterparts just don't need
to worry about such things. The topic of safer sex and condoms takes on a
whole different meaning when we speak of women. A man with a condom in
his wallet for that "special occasion" is praised as being a "player." However, in
some parts of the world a woman merely suggesting safer sex and condom use
may be subjected to abuse, both verbal and physical. A woman living with HIV
has additional issues she must be aware of and must deal with in order to have
a healthy life with HIV. We are going to discuss a couple of those issues here.

Pregnancy and HIV

At the outset of the epidemic, life after an HIV diagnosis was so short and so difficult that starting a family was out of the question. But as new, very effective HIV medications have come to market, life spans have become longer and life styles are approaching some semblance of normalcy. Today, having a family while living with HIV is not only possible, it occurs all the time. This is great news for couples having one or both partners infected with HIV. Planning and starting a family, however, is something that should not be taken lightly by anyone, HIV-positive or -negative. But for HIV-positive couples there are additional considerations that must be addressed before getting pregnant. Let's look at some of the issues facing HIV-positive couples who want to start a family.

Who Is the Positive Partner?

How couples approach starting a family depends largely on which partner is positive. There are unique issues to consider, depending on who is positive — the male or female member of the couple. Anytime serodiscordant partners (one positive and one negative partner) have sex, there is concern over HIV transmission from the positive partner to the negative. Typically, the answer is a simple one: safer sex — namely, using latex condoms during each sexual encounter. After all, condoms have been proven to be an extremely effective barrier to HIV transmission. Unfortunately, condoms have also been proven to be an effective barrier to pregnancy as well. So obviously, if the goal is pregnancy, latex condoms are not an option. The degree of HIV transmission risk depends primarily on which partner is positive. Let's look at a couple of different scenarios and what methods can be used to get pregnant, and at the same time minimizing the risk to the negative partner.

Positive Mother / Negative Father — The first possible scenario involves couples whose positive partner is the mother-to-be. Statistics have shown that the risk of HIV transmission from a woman to a man is less than the risk of transmission from a man to a woman. In fact, a woman's risk of being infected by a man during sex is eighteen times greater than a man's risk of being infected by a woman. But as low as the risk of transmission is, the risk is still there, and, in fact, transmission from women to men does occur. But there are ways to decrease that risk while still providing the opportunity for pregnancy.

- Outside of condom use, the best way to decrease the risk of HIV infection is to minimize the negative partner's exposure to active virus. By reducing the positive partner's HIV viral load, the negative partner's exposure to HIV is reduced and therefore the risk of infection is also reduced. This is accomplished by the use of HIV medications with the goal of suppressing HIV to an undetectable level. Keep in mind that while an undetectable viral load does reduce the risk of HIV transmission, it does not eliminate that risk entirely.

- It's also possible to reduce the risk of infection by treating the HIV-negative man with a post-exposure prophylaxis (PEP) regimen. In cases of rape or accidental exposure in the workplace, HIV medication regimens are prescribed in order to reduce the risk of infection. A study published in 1997 demonstrated that even using a post-exposure regimen of zidovudine (Retrovir, AZT) alone decreased HIV transmission by 79 percent. Studies as recent as 2007 confirmed these findings and showed multi-drug post-exposure prophylaxis regimens provided similar results. If used, PEP is taken for about four weeks post-exposure—or in this case, four weeks after unprotected sex with a positive female partner hoping to become pregnant.

Positive Father / Negative Mother —This scenario involves a positive man and a negative mother-to-be. As we mentioned in the previous section, the risk of HIV transmission from a man to a woman is much greater than from a woman to a man. But even in this scenario, there are ways to reduce the risk and allow these couples the opportunity to start a family.

- As is the case with a positive female, the risk of HIV transmission from a positive male partner to a negative female partner can be reduced by the use of HIV medications. Using HIV medications to suppress the virus to undetectable levels will reduce the risk of transmission to the negative partner significantly. Once again, even with an undetectable viral load, the HIV transmission risk is not eliminated entirely. However, the risk is diminished enough that couples trying to start a family are willing to accept that risk in exchange for the possibility of having a baby.
- Another option that is getting some attention is a procedure called *sperm washing*. Sperm washing is a technique that was first developed in Milan, Italy. The concept of sperm washing rests on the premise that HIV resides mainly in the seminal fluid (the thin liquid portion of the ejaculate) of an HIV-positive male. Sperm washing concentrates and separates the fertilizing sperm from the infectious seminal fluid. During ovulation, the woman is *artificially inseminated* (sperm is manually inserted into the uterus) with the concentrated sperm. Without the infectious seminal fluid, the theory is that the risk of the woman being infected with HIV is greatly reduced. Experts disagree on how well sperm washing protects the female. While the jury is still out regarding the effectiveness of the procedure, the clinic in Milan where the procedure was developed reports that after 2000 such sperm washing cases, there have been no HIV infections in the women they have artificially inseminated, and no children have been born HIV-infected. While it appears sperm washing is an effective option, potential problems do exist. Few, if any, medical insurance plans will cover sperm washing, and, unfortunately, the procedure is very expensive. Besides cost, another potential problem is that the procedure is not widely available. It

may be necessary to travel considerable distances to a facility offering the procedure, only adding to the already expensive price tag.

- The third option actually involves a third person. Specifically, the HIV-negative mother- to-be is artificially inseminated with donated sperm from an HIV-negative man. In most cases the sperm is obtained from an anonymous donor by way of a sperm bank. The couple does not know the donor of the sperm, and the donor does not know where his sperm was used. In some circumstances, a known donor can be used to impregnate the negative woman. For instance, a brother of the positive male partner may agree to donate the sperm that will be used to artificially inseminate the negative female partner or wife. The donor is sometimes referred to as a *surrogate*, meaning a substitute or stand-in. Keep in mind that there is widespread controversy surrounding artificial insemination. There have been cases of surrogates taking legal action in order to obtain visitation and parental rights after the baby is born. There also can be religious objections or ethical questions surrounding its use. Some see the procedure as unnatural or "tampering" with God's plan, while others view it as a gift that science has provided, allowing women who have trouble becoming pregnant to experience the joy of having children.

- Another option used to decrease the HIV transmission risk is post-exposure prophylaxis (PEP). Just as people who have been accidentally exposed to HIV take PEP to reduce the risk of infection, women can take PEP after having unprotected sex in an attempt to get pregnant. Caution must be used when prescribing PEP because there are HIV medications that can cause harm to an unborn child.

- Some clinics have been experimenting with pre-exposure prophylaxis: taking a dose of HIV medication prior to having unprotected sex in hopes of decreasing the risk of HIV transmission. Studies have been done using the drug tenofovir (Viread) because of its rapid uptake into the blood stream. In this case the drug is to be taken two hours prior to unprotected intercourse. Consult your HIV specialist or fertility specialist to find out what options are available and are best for you.

Positive Mother / Positive Father — You may think that because both partners in this scenario are HIV-positive there is nothing to consider. Actually, there are a couple of issues that have to be addressed. First, keep in mind that even though both partners are positive, the issue of HIV re-infection must be considered. If you recall, earlier in this text we discussed HIV re-infection. To summarize, an HIV-positive person can be re-infected with another strain of HIV when having unprotected sex with his or her HIV-positive partner. This can make treating the HIV in the re-infected partner much more difficult. So when trying to start a family, the couple with two positive partners should only have unprotected sex during the female's time of ovulation — that time when the female is most likely to get pregnant. During other times of the month, and after conception has occurred, the couple with two positive partners should return to using condoms to prevent HIV re-infection.

The other consideration is that once conception has occurred it is absolutely imperative that the pregnant partner get into prenatal care as soon as possible. Even if she was not on HIV medications prior to becoming pregnant, she will be placed on HIV medications during pregnancy in order to decrease the risk of infecting her unborn child. After delivery, the new mother may be able to stop her medications if she was not taking any prior to her pregnancy. But to re-emphasize, once pregnant, the mother-to-be must get into prenatal care as soon as possible for the health of her baby.

Other Risk Reduction Methods for Discordant Couples Trying to Have a Baby

Along with the options we have just discussed, there are other risk reduction methods that will make it possible for discordant couples to start the family they have been dreaming of while at the same time keeping each partner as safe and healthy as possible.

- Prior to starting a family, both partners should be tested for sexually transmitted diseases (STDs). Any active STDs should be treated prior to getting pregnant. Because the presence of STDs can increase the risk of HIV transmission to the negative partner, any STDs should be treated as soon as possible.
- Couples should only have unprotected sex during the woman's most fertile time of the month (during ovulation) when the chance of pregnancy is highest. While ovulation varies from woman to woman, it is typically about ten to fourteen days after your menstrual period ends. Safer sex methods should be used during the rest of the month and after conception (pregnancy) occurs.
- Couples should avoid "dry sex" (sex with little or no lubrication). Friction can cause small tears or irritation to the vaginal tissue, which opens portals that allow HIV to enter the bloodstream. Also avoid the use of any lubricating products that could irritate the mucosa of the vagina for the same reason; tissue irritation increases the risk of HIV infection.

Preventing Mother-to-Child HIV Transmission

HIV can spread from a woman to her baby in two ways—during pregnancy and delivery, and during breastfeeding. Without interventions, *vertical transmission* (transmission from an infected pregnant woman to her unborn child) is very efficient—about one in four births. Exposure to the infected blood and amniotic fluid while in the uterus or during a vaginal delivery is the route by which HIV enters the baby's bloodstream. The longer the baby is exposed to these fluids the higher the risk of infection. But there are methods used today that have succeeded in virtually eliminating the risk of vertical transmission.

- HIV medication regimens are given to the mother during pregnancy and during delivery in hopes of bringing her HIV viral load to an undetectable level. The lower the viral load the lower the risk of transmission.
- Typically, in those women with detectable viral loads, the child is delivered using a cesarean section (C-section), thereby reducing the amount of time the baby is exposed to the fluids of delivery. For those women with undetectable viral loads, vaginal delivery is sometimes considered.
- After delivery, an HIV regimen is prescribed for the newborn. Typically treatment consists of the drug *zidovudine* (Retrovir, AZT) that begins after delivery and continues for about six weeks.

Another route of HIV infection in newborns is breastfeeding. In fact, breastfeeding carries an extremely high risk of transmission — somewhere between 25 and 30 percent. Because of the high risk, HIV-positive mothers are cautioned not to breast feed or manually express breast milk to feed their baby. Instead, commercial formulas should be used. In parts of the world where clean water and alternatives to breast milk are readily available, this is not a problem. However, in less developed countries, such as countries in Africa, breastfeeding may be the only option. Scientists are researching ways to reduce the risk of HIV infection from breastfeeding. Recently studies suggest that placing the mother on the drug nevirapine (Viramune) after delivery provides protection for the baby during breastfeeding. While the recommendation is still to avoid breastfeeding when possible, research is making breastfeeding safer in those circumstances where it is the only option.

Final Considerations for Discordant Couples Trying to Get Pregnant

Before taking that big step and getting pregnant, there are a few items discordant couples need to consider. While these issues should not deter efforts to become parents, couples must understand the potential barriers and risks associated with pregnancy.

- Realizing that trying to start a family can put the negative partner at risk and can affect sexual spontaneity, sexual drive, and the ability to conceive. Experts believe that stress related to concerns of HIV infection can affect a woman's likelihood to conceive or a partner's desire to have sex at all.
- It's possible that the positive partner will eventually have health-related issues that could impact his or her ability to parent a child. These types of health concerns can affect the couple's desire to have sex and their ability to conceive.

• Despite measures that minimize the risk of having an HIV-infected baby, there is still the possibility, however small, that the newborn could be HIV-infected. The stress of that possibility can cause relationship issues and diminish the desire to start a family.

• Depending on available resources, not all measures that reduce the HIV risk to negative partners will be available. For instance, sperm washing and artificial insemination reduce transmission risk, but because these methods are not covered by insurance, they may not be available to couples with limited resources.

WOMEN STAYING HEALTHY

HIV-positive people face many issues that can in some way jeopardize their health. From medication side effects to AIDS-related weight loss, people with HIV are at risk for a variety of conditions, illnesses and infections. However, HIV-positive women face all these issues and more, issues only they as women face each and every day. In fact, there is evidence that women are more vulnerable to HIV and the conditions that accompany the virus. So why is that the case?

Physical Differences

The incidence of heterosexual transmission in the United States has been on the rise since 1985. At that time, about three percent of all known cases were heterosexually transmitted. That figure today is about 27 percent. What's more, 70 percent of all new HIV infections are a result of heterosexual transmission; worldwide, that figure is closer to 90 percent. And, unfortunately, it's women who bear the greatest risk — due mostly to their anatomy. The vagina is lined with very fragile and highly vascular mucosal tissue. Women are especially susceptible to heterosexual transmission because that mucosal lining offers a large surface area that is exposed to HIV-infected seminal fluid during unprotected sex. In addition, because vaginal tissue is so fragile, small tears can form during intercourse, creating portals of entry that allow HIV to reach the bloodstream. These factors are what make infection from men to women easier than from women to men.

Gender Inequities

Especially in developing countries, prevailing gender inequities leads to higher-risk behaviors. For instance, in many cultures women are not free to refuse sex or to insist on safer sex. In fact, in some parts of the world women are subjected to violence or rape by merely suggesting condom use. Many cultures assume women are prostitutes or are promiscuous for simply having a condom in their possession or for suggesting the use of safer sex practices. And as unbelievable as it may sound, in some parts of the world possession of condoms by women is actually a criminal offense. In these cultures and societies, men assume a position of power and control over women, minimizing the amount of input women have when deciding whether or not to use safer sex practices. In addition, women have less access to employment and education in these developing countries. Often, the sex trade is the only option for women trying to earn money to feed their children. And, sadly, sexual violence against women is very high in some areas, exposing these women to high-risk behaviors with multiple partners, all without their consent.

Increased Risk of Illness

Women have an increased risk of reproductive illnesses, including vaginal yeast infections, pelvic inflammatory disease (PID), and cervical cancer, as a result of Human Papillomavirus (HPV) infection. The presence of sexually transmitted diseases significantly increases the risk of HIV infection.

No Resources / No Insurance

Because women often have lower incomes than men or work in jobs that offer minimal benefits, they have less access to affordable medical insurance and therefore HIV care. Without a means to pay for healthcare or medications, women are more likely to postpone trips to their doctors, or will not fill their HIV medication prescriptions. What's more, because women lack transportation (more so than men), they will often miss appointments with their HIV specialist or gynecologist. And, as we know, without regular healthcare it's difficult to maintain your health.

Family First

Women tend to assume more family care responsibilities than do men. Because of this, women are more likely to sacrifice their own healthcare in order to care for their family, especially their children. In fact, it's not uncommon for women to sacrifice their own health for the sake of their children. For instance, in situations of limited resources, mothers will stop their medications so they can afford the medicines for their children. And it's not uncommon for a mother to forego her own doctor's appointment in order to get her child to theirs. Simply put, mothers see themselves as less important than the rest of their family. When push comes to shove, a mom will always put the needs of her family above her own needs.

OPPORTUNISTIC INFECTIONS
UNIQUE TO HIV-POSITIVE WOMEN

As we learned in an earlier chapter, being infected with HIV places you at risk for a variety of associated conditions and illnesses. While women are subject to the same group of conditions as men, there are some conditions and diseases that are unique to women. These conditions jeopardize a woman's health and in some cases can jeopardize a woman's life. Let's look at several of those conditions that can be a serious threat to a woman's health.

Pelvic Inflammatory Disease (PID)

Pelvic inflammatory disease is actually a group of infections that affect the female reproductive system — specifically, the vagina, cervix, uterus, fallopian tubes and ovaries. While chlamydia and gonorrhea are the common infectious organisms, various other organisms can lead to PID, including tuberculosis and various bacterial infections. The difference between PID in HIV-positive women and HIV-negative women is not well documented, but there have been studies that attempt to identify the differences. One such study found that HIV-positive women were more likely to require surgical intervention as a result of PID — necessary because of damage caused by the infection. Also, HIV-infected women were more likely to develop an abscess (pocket of infection) as a result of PID. Thankfully, the study also showed that HIV-positive women responded to antibiotics just as well as their HIV-negative counterparts. While this study, and ones like it, did show PID can be aggressive in HIV-positive women, whether it needs to be treated more aggressively in HIV-infected women is still unclear.

The classic signs and symptoms of PID include severe abdominal pain, pelvic pain, vaginal discharge, and fever. Oddly, in women living with HIV, PID can often be silent, exhibiting no signs or symptoms at all. However, even in the absence of symptoms, PID in the HIV-positive woman can advance quickly, leading to the formation of fallopian tube abscesses. These abscesses, if left untreated, can result in sterility or, in severe cases, can be fatal.

Treatment of PID consists of antibiotics, either oral or intravenous (given directly into a vein), depending on the severity of the infection. In fact, severe infections may require hospitalization and both oral and intravenous antibiotics.

TABLE 11. PELVIC INFLAMMATORY DISEASE

Signs and Symptoms
- Some women have no symptoms at all
- Severe abdominal pain
- Pelvic pain
- Vaginal discharge
- Fever

Treatment
- Treatment varies depending on severity of the infection.
- Antibiotics are given orally or intravenously, depending again on the severity of infection.
- Severe infections may require both oral and intravenous antibiotics and hospitalization.

Vaginal Yeast Infections

We have seen that oral yeast infections ("thrush") are very common in men and women living with HIV. Another type of yeast infection, the vaginal yeast infection, is common in HIV-positive and -negative women alike. And while this type of fungal infection is easily treated in negative women, the infection can be more frequent, more severe and much more difficult to treat in HIV-positive women. In fact, chronic and frequent vaginal yeast infections can be an early sign of HIV.

Symptoms of chronic yeast infections include thick white to yellow vaginal discharge; foul odor, pain, burning, and/or itching of the vaginal area; and white or gray patches on the vagina. Once again, these symptoms are difficult to effectively treat in HIV-positive women, and with each recurrence the symptoms often become more severe.

HIV-negative women can usually treat their vaginal yeast infections with as little as a single dose of prescription-strength oral antifungal medication. In fact, some yeast infections in negative women can be treated with as little as an over-the-counter antifungal cream. Positive women, on the other hand, struggle with frequent, recurrent vaginal yeast infections that seldom are able to be treated with a single-dose medication or an over-the-counter cream. Depending on the severity of the infection, the treatment of choice is typically oral antifungal medications taken over a three to ten day period. However, in cases of severe or recurrent infections, it may take multiple courses of antifungal medication to completely resolve a yeast infection in an HIV-positive woman.

The best way to treat a yeast infection is to prevent it from occurring in the first place. There are simple things you can do to reduce the frequency and severity of yeast infections. These include eating yogurt that contains activated bacterial cultures, as well as decreasing the amount of sugar in your diet. Both of these simple steps make it harder for vaginal yeast to grow and flourish. One thing to keep in mind is that yeast infections can be passed between sexual partners, so sex should be avoided during active yeast infections.

TABLE 12. VAGINAL YEAST INFECTION

Signs and Symptoms
- Caused by a fungal infection
- Thick white or yellow vaginal discharge
- Foul vaginal odor
- Vaginal pain, burning or itching
- White or gray patches on and around the vagina

Treatment
- Treatment varies, depending on severity of the infection, and is typically oral or topical.
- In HIV-negative women treatment can be as little as one dose of medication.
- Treatment is typically a 3–10 day course of antifungal medications.
- HIV-positive women may need multiple course of antifungal medication to completely resolve the infection.

Bacterial Vaginosis

While somewhat similar to vaginal yeast infections, bacterial vaginosis differs in that it is caused by a bacterium, while yeast infections are caused by a fungus. Spread during unsafe sex, vaginosis is characterized by foul smelling, frothy vaginal discharge. There are available treatments for bacterial vaginosis; however, treatment for HIV-positive women sometimes requires a longer course of medication. In HIV-negative women treatment with the antibiotic metronidazole (Flagyl), taken twice a day for seven days, usually clears the infection. However, HIV-positive women sometimes need to take a second course of antibiotic to completely clear the infection. For those women who have a hard time taking oral medications, there are topical antibiotic creams that can be used. However, this type of treatment typically is not effective for HIV-positive women. One thing to keep in mind is that since vaginosis can be sexually transmitted to other women, female sexual partners of women with vaginosis must be treated as well. Also, sexual toys such as vibrators or "dildos" should not be shared and should be washed thoroughly between uses.

TABLE 13. BACTERIAL VAGINOSIS

Signs and Symptoms
- Caused by a bacterial infection
- Foul vaginal odor
- Frothy vaginal discharge
- Infection is sexually transmitted from one woman to another, so partners of women with the infection should be treated as well
- Sex toys should not be shared, especially when symptoms are present

Treatment
- Treatment for HIV-positive women requires a longer course than that for HIV-negative women.
- Treatment is administered typically twice a day for 7 days using the medication metronidazole (Flagyl).
- HIV-positive women usually need a second course of treatment to completely resolve infection.
- Topical antibiotics may be used in some cases.

Trichomonas

One final type of vaginal infection common in HIV-positive women is called trichomonas. This vaginal infection is caused by a protozoa, a large group of one-cell microscopic organisms that can cause infection in people living with HIV. This infection is characterized by a large amount of thick, green or yellow vaginal discharge, accompanied by pain, soreness, and severe vaginal itching. In women with normal immune systems, about 95 percent of these infections can be successfully treated with a single two-gram dose of the antibiotic metronidazole (Flagyl). On the other hand, women with weakened immune systems, including those with HIV, typically need to be treated for seven days with a twice-daily dose (375 milligrams) of metronidazole (Flagyl) to clear the infection. Like bacterial vaginosis, all sex partners should be treated to prevent recurrence and to stop the spread of trichomonas to other people.

TABLE 14. TRICHOMONAS

Signs and Symptoms
- Caused by a single-cell organism known as a protozoa
- Characterized by a large amount of thick, green or yellow vaginal discharge
- Vaginal pain, soreness, and itching

Treatment
- In women with a normal immune system, 95% can be treated with a single 2-gram dose of metronidazole.
- Women with HIV need to be treated with seven days of twice-daily metronidazole.
- All sex partners should be treated to prevent recurrence and the spread of trichomonas to others.

HEALTH SCREENING—THE IMPORTANCE OF PAP TESTS

The *Papanicolaou Test*, more commonly known as the *Pap Test* or *Pap Smear*, is an important health screening tool for all women, HIV-positive and -negative alike. Specifically, the pap test is the best screening tool available for the early detection of cervical cancer. For HIV-positive women the importance of regular pap tests can't be overstated. In fact, HIV and gynecology experts alike agree that teaching women about the importance of pap tests should be part of every HIV education program. Positive women must understand the importance of the pap test as an essential part of a complete health screening program.

TABLE 15. CERVICAL CANCER SCREENING GUIDELINES— HIV-NEGATIVE WOMAN

When to start having pap tests	3 years after first episode of intercourse but no later than the age of 21 years
How often conventional pap tests should be done	Initially should be done once per year. Can be done every 2–3 years for women older than 30 who have had 3 negative tests
How often thin prep pap tests should be done	Initially should be done once per year. Can be done every 2–3 years for women older than 30 who have had 3 negative tests
How often if HPV testing is used	Every 3 years of HPV and the cell cytology is negative
When to stop having pap tests	Women older than 70 years with 3 recent and consecutive tests, and no positive tests in the last 10 years
Post–total hysterectomy	Discontinue for benign reasons and no history of high grade CIN lesions.

What Is a Pap Test?

Gynecologists, doctors that specialize in the treatment of female reproductive diseases, use the pap test to examine cells of the cervix. The cervix is the most distal part of the uterus and is located at the point where the uterus and vagina come together. Gynecologists examine cells of the cervix for changes that may indicate cancer or precancerous conditions. Because cells of the cervix are prone to cancerous and precancerous changes, frequent examination of these cells is indicated. And because HIV-positive women are at an increased risk for cervical cancer, pap tests every six to twelve months are absolutely essential. Typically, the first two pap tests will be done six months apart. If both are negative, the HIV-positive woman can then have paps every twelve months. If either of the first two are positive for an abnormality, then the HIV-positive woman must have her paps every six months.

By using the pap test and examining cervical cells regularly, gynecologists are able to detect any cellular changes that occur, allowing steps to be taken to treat those cells before they become cancerous or before any cancer spreads to other parts of the body. This is important because early detection of cancer cells and precancerous cells allows for earlier treatment, and studies have proven this translates to a better prognosis for the woman.

How Is a Pap Test Done?

A Pap test is typically done as part of a routine pelvic exam. The gynecologist visually examines the external parts of the female reproductive system — namely, the external anatomy of the vagina — looking for lesions, genital warts, or other abnormalities. To examine the inside of the vagina, an instrument called a speculum is inserted and opened slowly, spreading the entrance of the vagina, allowing the gynecologist to see the vaginal walls and cervix. Again, the gynecologist is looking for lesions, vaginal discharge, irritation, masses, or bleeding. After the visual examination of the vagina and cervix, a pap test is done.

Examining the cells of the cervix requires a cell sample be sent to the lab. To collect the cells, a long cotton-tip swab is inserted into the vagina and wiped against the cervix. When the swab comes in contact with the cervix, cells adhere to the cotton tip. The swab containing the cells is placed in a special solution that preserves the cells until they can be examined in the lab. Once in the lab, specially trained lab technologists examine the cells under a microscope, looking to identify any changes in cellular structure that may indicate disease. If abnormal cells are identified, the results are reported to the physician, and further follow-up will be necessary.

What Do the Results of the Pap Test Mean?

Typically, most HIV-negative women will have a normal pap test, meaning the cells collected from the cervix show no signs of structural change. If this is the case, nothing more has to be done except schedule your next pap test, typically for one year later. However, HIV-positive women seem to have a higher incidence of abnormal pap tests. In other words, the cells collected during the pap test show some degree of structural change. These changes are classified in one of several categories, based on the type and degree of structural changes that are present. These classifications are:

- **Mild, Moderate, or Severe Dysplasia (abnormal growth)**—These cells have undergone changes, but those changes are not yet cancerous. They can also be referred to as *"atypia squamous cells of undetermined significance"* (ASCUS). However, these cells may become cancerous if left untreated. Therefore, more frequent monitoring is required, and eventually treatment may be necessary. These changes can be caused by inflammation or infection. Depending on how extensive these changes are, your doctor will do another pap test in six months.

- **Squamous Intraepithelial Lesion (SIL)**—These are abnormal cells found only on the surface of the cervix. The cellular changes can range from low-grade (LSIL) to high-grade (HSIL) and can indicate the presence of cancer.

- **Cervical Intraepithelial Neoplasm (CIN)**—This is another way to describe abnormal cells on the surface of the cervix. The cells that have undergone the most severe changes are those that can be cancerous or become cancerous over time if left untreated. Depending on how much of the cervix contains these types of cells, they are classified as CIN 1, CIN 2, or the most extensive, CIN 3.

- **Carcinoma In-Situ**—This describes cells that have changed and become cancerous. They only affect the surface layers, but left untreated can migrate deeper into the cervical tissue, resulting in cervical cancer. You may see these results referred to as HSIL or CIN 3. Left untreated, cervical cancer can be fatal.

- **Cervical Cancer**—These results indicate that cancer has already migrated deep into the cervix. This result will require further, more invasive testing, chemotherapy treatment, radiation therapy, and/or possibly surgery to remove the areas of cancer.

TABLE 16. WHAT DO YOUR PAP RESULTS MEAN?

Atypia Squamous Cells of Undetermined Significance (ASCUS)
(Mild, moderate or severe dysplasia)

- These cells have begun to undergo abnormal changes, but those changes are not yet considered cancerous.
- These changes can become cancerous if ignored.
- More frequent monitoring is indicated, typically every 6 months.
- These changes are typically due to inflammation or infection.

Squamous Intraepithelial Lesion (SIL)
(Low-grade / LSIL to high grade / HSIL)
- These abnormal cells are found only on the surface of the cervix.
- The degree of abnormality ranges from low grade (LSIL) to high grade (HSIL).
- This can indicate the presence of cancer.

Cervical Intraepithelial Neoplasm (CIN)
(Ranges from CIN 1 to CIN 3)
- CIN 1— One-third of the surface of the cervix has abnormal cells (mildly abnormal cells).
- CIN 2 — Two-thirds of the surface of the cervix has abnormal cells (moderately abnormal cells).
- CIN 3 — The entire surface of the cervix has abnormal cells (severely abnormal cells); sometimes called *carcinoma in situ*.

Carcinoma in situ
(HSIL or CIN 3)
- Sometimes referred to as HSIL or CIN 3.
- Left untreated, carcinoma in situ can be fatal.

Cervical Cancer
- These results indicate a condition where cancerous cells have already migrated deep into the cervix.
- This requires more invasive testing (biopsy), chemotherapy treatment, radiation therapy, and possibly surgery to remove the cancerous areas.

HPV AND CERVICAL CANCER IN HIV-POSITIVE WOMEN

In an earlier chapter we learned that Human Papillomavirus (HPV) is a very common sexually transmitted virus. About 45 percent of all 20 to 24 year olds have HPV infection. But as common as it is in the general population, it is even more common in HIV-positive women. One study indicated that greater than 85 percent of HIV-positive women have cervical HPV infection. And while the typical HIV-negative woman has an immune system strong enough to fight off most HPV complications, most HIV-positive women tend to have more persistent HPV. In other words, HIV-positive women are more likely to develop abnormal cellular changes of the cervix, which in turn can progress to cancer much faster. Even after treatment, the rate of recurrence in HIV-positive women is higher than in the general population. Because HPV tends to be more aggressive in HIV-positive women, and because the risk of cervical cancer as a result of HPV infection is high, regularly scheduled pap tests are an absolute must.

Our Final Lap

Medical issues associated with HIV are numerous. Vaginal yeast infections, genital herpes, lymphoma and invasive cervical cancer are only a few of the medical complications associated with the disease. But there are other non-medical issues that accompany HIV that can make life difficult for positive men and women alike. Social issues, including prejudice, discrimination, and isolation, are common. Practical issues, such as traveling with prescription medications or restricted travel due to an HIV diagnosis, can make life very complicated for any positive person whose job or recreation includes travel. Finally, deciding who will care for your children or make your financial decisions if you are unable to make them yourself can wear heavily on the emotional state of people living with HIV. We conclude our educational journey through this text with information that will help you deal with the practical side of HIV. The following issues are among the most common that affect your day to day life when living with HIV.

Legal / Ethical Issues Faced by HIV-Positive People

As this text has demonstrated, HIV infection presents a variety of challenges for those infected. Some are medical in nature — the dangers of opportunistic infections, for instance. Some are psychological, such as the emotional challenges resulting from an HIV diagnosis. And finally, some issues can be social in nature — dating for the first time after diagnosis, to name just one. All these challenges can make for a complicated and sometimes difficult life. And if those issues weren't enough, legal and ethical issues seem to crop up fairly often in the lives of many HIV-positive people; being fired unjustly, denied an apartment, or losing medical insurance have all been known to occur as an indirect result of HIV. So what are some of the most common issues, and what can be done to make them more manageable?

DISCRIMINATION AND PREJUDICE

Since the earliest days of the epidemic, people living with HIV and AIDS have been subjected to discrimination and prejudice at almost every turn. By misunderstanding the true nature of HIV, those without the disease become afraid — afraid of that which they don't understand. Their fear is directed outward toward those suffering the ill effects of the virus, adding to the issues HIV introduces into day-to-day life. Simply put, instead of helping those living with the disease, the fearful and ignorant turn away, creating an atmosphere of prejudice, isolation, and discrimination for those trying to live a healthy and normal live in the face of some pretty big odds.

Don't for a minute believe this sort of ignorance and insensitivity is unique to the lay person. When the epidemic first emerged, experts identified groups of people they felt were at increased risk of acquiring the new infection. Gay men were one such group. So high was the risk that experts referred to the new infectious disease as "*GRID*," meaning "gay-related immunodeficiency," insinuating that being gay somehow was responsible for HIV. Some even referred to the new infection as *"gay cancer."* In response to these labels, lay people passed judgment upon gay men, suggesting they were the true cause of HIV and its rapid spread.

Thankfully, those labels were abandoned many years ago, replaced with the terms HIV and AIDS. However, the public perception that HIV and being gay go hand in hand is, for the most part, alive and well. Realizing people still associate homosexuality with HIV and AIDS, infected people fear they will become the target of hatred and prejudice. They fear more than anything that their diagnosis will somehow become public knowledge, which could lead to mistreatment, discrimination, or in some cases violence and physical harm. And their fears are not unfounded. People have lost jobs, their insurance, and their homes as a result of their HIV status. Sure, there are "official" reasons behind these occurrences, but we all know that an HIV diagnosis plays an "unofficial" role. But fortunately, legislators have recognized the struggles some HIV-positive people have to endure just to feed their family or put a roof over their head. Legal measures have been taken to protect HIV-positive people from the mistreatment of others. Understanding the legal resources you have at your disposal is an important way to protect yourself from the fear and ignorance of others.

The Americans with Disabilities Act (ADA)

Fortunately, experts in the field of HIV, as well as enlightened members of our government, have recognized the issues faced by HIV-infected people and have taken steps to protect them. One such step is voting to designate HIV and AIDS as a disability. By doing so, HIV-positive people are able to benefit from the protective umbrella of the *Americans with Disabilities Act* (ADA). The ADA provides civil rights protection to people living with disabilities. Persons living with HIV, whether they are symptomatic or not, are considered to have a disability that significantly impairs their daily lives. Because of this fact they are protected by the ADA.

The legal precedence for this decision involves the case of an asymptomatic HIV-positive woman whose dentist refused to fill her decayed tooth, claiming the woman needed to have the procedure done at a hospital because of risks associated with her HIV. The woman disagreed, believing that the dentist's decision was based on fear for himself and not on what was best for her as his patient. She felt being forced to take on the extra cost of a hospital visit was unjust. So she filed a lawsuit against the dentist, citing the ADA as the basis of her civil complaint. The dentist contended that because the woman was asymptomatic she should not be protected by the ADA. In other words, the dentist felt that because the woman was not symptomatic she could not be considered disabled and therefore could not be protected by the ADA. The courts disagreed, and from that point forward, HIV-positive people, symptomatic and asymptomatic alike, have been protected by the ADA.

In addition to protecting the civil rights of the disabled, the ADA also guarantees equal opportunity for employment; equal access to state and local government services, transportation, and telecommunications; and equal access to public accommodations such as hotels, hospitals, restaurants, and housing.

Public Accommodations—The ADA assures that people with disabilities, including people living with HIV, have access to public accommodations. In other words, people can't be deprived of such things as employment, housing, access to health care, or admission to restaurants or hotels due to their disability. In addition, reasonable accommodations must be made for those people with disabilities, allowing them to access these public services. Reasonable accommodations are defined as, but not limited to:

- making employee facilities usable by those employees with disabilities; for example, installing amplified telephones for those employees that are hard of hearing;
- job and schedule restructuring or reassignment to a position better suited to the person and his or her disability;
- acquiring or modifying equipment, devices, policies, or training material in an effort to accommodate the disabled employee;
- providing qualified readers or interpreters for those employees who are unable to read or who speak a language other than English.

For example, public places must have wheelchair accessible restroom facilities for those people confined to a wheelchair. The ADA also prevents doctors, hospitals, and dentists from categorically refusing to treat HIV-positive patients due to "public health concerns." The exception to that rule is that doctors can refuse to treat patients outside of their specialty, meaning that an orthopedic surgeon can refuse to treat HIV because infectious disease is not their specialty. Instead, they refer such patients to a specialist—in the case or our example, an HIV specialist.

Employment—Part of the protection offered through the ADA is the right to equal employment opportunities. The ADA protects people with disabilities from being discriminated against in the workplace. For instance, the ADA prohibits employers from not hiring a person with HIV because they fear that person will be sick in the future. In fact, having HIV without complications is almost never a valid reason not to deny employment. Furthermore, an employer can't require a medical exam before making a job offer, but can make an offer contingent upon passing a medical exam if a medical exam is required by all people in that job category. Keep in mind that if you request accommodations under the umbrella of the ADA, your medical condition may come into question, which may jeopardize your confidentiality. While you are not obligated in any way to disclose your HIV status, you may have to do so if you are asking for accommodations under the ADA. You will be required to prove your disability in order to access the benefits and protections offered by the ADA, which will require you to divulge your diagnosis. Your employer must be aware of your HIV diagnosis in order to make "reasonable accommodations" surrounding your job. Once your employer is aware of your disability, he or she is obligated to make "reasonable accommodations" that allow you to perform your job. For example, if you have peripheral neuropathy in your hands that makes it difficult to use a mouse, your employer must provide you with a special type of mouse designed to minimize the symptoms of neuropathy (e.g., a trackball).

Insurance — The ADA prevents employers from denying insurance coverage to disabled employees or from charging increased insurance premiums based on a disability. In fact, the ADA prohibits employers from entering into contracts with any insurance company that discriminates based on a disability. Keep in mind that insurance companies are permitted to utilize a preexisting condition clause when issuing insurance to an employee. This means that if you have a preexisting illness (e.g., HIV) at the time of being hired, any claims related to that illness will not be reimbursed if they occur before the expiration of a waiting period (most often between six months and one year after hiring). Keep in mind that this preexisting clause can only be included if it is applied to all employees with preexisting conditions, not just those with HIV.

Ways to Fight Discrimination

If you feel you are being discriminated against due to your HIV diagnosis, there are avenues you can pursue to fight for your rights and for equal and fair treatment. Your first step is to contact your local ADA office to file a complaint. The telephone number can be found in the government section of your telephone book. Keep in mind you must file your complaint with the ADA within 180 days of the alleged discrimination. Another thing to keep in mind when taking on your fight is that your diagnosis and medical history will most likely come into the public light. In fact, every aspect of your work record, attendance history and private life in general will come into question. Any privacy you had will probably be lost to some degree. Depending on who you name in your complaint, it could be a very stressful fight. Regardless, discrimination needs to be fought, and the ADA is there to protect you.

Legal Assistance — As we all know, hiring an attorney can be very costly. Unless you have a very good job, hiring a private lawyer to assist with your legal issues will be very difficult. However, most large cities have lawyers and law practices that assist people on fixed incomes or with limited resources. To find these law practices or individual lawyers, contact the State Bar Association in your state. You can find their telephone number in your local directory or search the internet for the Bar Association in your state.

One more thing to keep in mind when seeking out an attorney is to find a lawyer familiar with issues associated with HIV. For example, find an attorney that is experienced in the ADA and what it offers HIV-infected people. Just as you would choose a doctor specializing in broken bones to fix your broken leg, you should choose a lawyer that specializes in HIV issues. And while it may be expensive, there are government and private funds available to offset some of the cost. Many times, if you have a case, an attorney will represent you with the understanding that their fee will be paid out of the final financial settlement, if there is one. You may even come across a lawyer that will donate their time, depending on your case and situation. Obviously, there are limits to this sort of service, and it should not be expected from all practices or attorneys. When you find an attorney to represent you, make sure they outline their fee schedules and requirements at your first visit.

ADVANCED DIRECTIVES

Whether we are healthy or sick, we all think about our own mortality from time to time. Most of us fear death to some degree, so much so, in fact, that we push it aside and choose to think about it another day. Like so much of our life, our death and circumstances surrounding that death are out of our control. However, there are ways to regain some control over certain aspects of our death and how it impacts survivors. *Advanced directives* are legal documents that allow us to maintain some control over end-of-life issues in hopes of making our death as "good" as possible and to minimize the impact our death has on survivors. Advanced directives allow us to make our end-of-life wishes known ahead of time in case we are unable to do so later. While it is very important to have an advance directive in place, there are a few questions you should first consider before having your attorney draw up the papers.

- Who would you like to make your personal decisions in the event you are unable to make them for yourself?
- If you become unconscious, become senile, or are diagnosed with a terminal illness that will likely end your life within six months, do you want to be placed on life-prolonging measures such as mechanical breathing machines (ventilators), drugs, feeding tubes, or resuscitation (CPR)?
- What type of medications are you willing to take, and to what extent would you like to be treated, if you suffer a stroke or other catastrophic event that makes you totally dependant on others for your daily care?
- What sort of physical, mental, and social abilities do you consider essential for a good quality of life?
- Do you want to receive all treatments recommended by your physicians and other members of your treatment team?

Is an Attorney Necessary to Write Your Advanced Directives?

You can use an attorney if you wish to prepare your advanced directives, but it's not necessary. If you choose not to use an attorney, there are a few things you want to make certain of prior to signing any documents. First, make certain that you discuss your intent with the person you name on the advanced directive prior to drawing up the document. Make certain they will be able to make difficult decisions in the event you become incompetent, unconscious, or terminally ill. Second, remember that your advanced directive needs to have a witness signature along with your signature. The law prohibits a family member, the person you name in the directive, your attorney, or any member of your health care team to act as a witness for your advanced directives.

Durable Power of Attorney — The unpleasant reality of any chronic disease, HIV included, is that eventually illness may make it difficult or impossible for you to make rational decisions regarding your health care, finances, or legal issues. There is a legal document that can benefit those people who are unable to make decisions due to illness. A *durable power of attorney* is a document that legally gives another person the power to make personal decisions for you in the event you are unable to make them yourself. In other words, it is a document that allows someone to speak on your behalf in times when you are unable to speak for yourself. When you ("the principal") sign a durable power of attorney, another person ("the agent") will have the legal ability to make decisions for you. Typically, the powers are broad, covering just about any decision or act that you make regarding your personal affairs. One exception is that the power of attorney does not give the agent the right to change or revoke your will. While some durable powers of attorney take effect or remain in effect regardless of the principal's mental status, those related to health care issues typically include clauses stating that the power of attorney only takes effect in the event the principal becomes mentally incapacitated.

LIVING WILLS

A living will is one of the most widely known advanced directives. Simply put, a living will allows you to refuse medical treatment in the case of terminal illness. For instance, a person dying of cancer can have a living will that states he or she does not want to have any heroic life-saving procedures. For example, a living will can state you do not want to be placed on a mechanical breathing machine in order to prolong life. Simply put, a living will allows the terminally ill (death expected in six months or less) to legally refuse any life support measures. While the living will is useful in the face of terminal illness, there are situations where a durable power of attorney is better suited.

- Living wills are not valid in all states. Check with your state to see if a living will has legal standing where you live.
- Living wills are valid only in the case of terminal illness. A durable power of attorney applies to any illness.
- A living will only allows you to refuse treatment, whereas a durable power

of attorney allows you to accept, refuse, or withdraw different forms of treatment.

• Unlike the durable power of attorney, a living will does not allow you to appoint a person to make decisions for you in the event you become unable to make those decisions for yourself.

Stand-By Guardianship Order

Most of us don't cherish the thought of having someone care for our children. But what happens if an illness makes you temporarily unable to care for them yourself? Most people would want to choose who cares for their children in that situation. A *stand-by guardianship order* is a legal document that allows you to designate who will care for your children if you are unable. The document assigns temporary legal guardianship to the person or persons of your choice, and only takes effect in the event you become unable to care for the children on your own. The document typically has to be renewed every sixty days. There are permanent guardianship orders that will assign permanent decision-making rights to the person of your choice, and in the process sacrifice your own parental and guardianship rights. A permanent guardianship order is typically only used in the case of your permanent incapacitation or death. In times of temporary incapacitation, a stand-by guardianship order is sufficient.

Traveling with HIV

Since the tragedy of 9/11, security measures associated with travel are tighter than ever before. More stringent policies regarding what can be carried onto an airplane, cruise ship, or train has made traveling with prescription medications much more difficult. Also, the stigma associated with an HIV diagnosis can make travel outside the United States complicated. While most people will have little difficulty traveling with HIV, some will have problems, especially if they are not properly prepared. Let's look at some traveling tips that will make your vacation carefree.

Traveling with Prescription Medication

Throughout this text it has been repeatedly stressed that taking your medicines each and every day is important if you are to stay healthy and your HIV medications are to be effective. Even missing one or two days' worth of doses can ultimately lead to viral mutation, eventually necessitating a medication change. So when you are traveling it's important to make sure your medications travel with you. Here are some ideas that will make traveling with your medications much easier.

Anticipate What You Will Need — Before leaving on your trip, assess how much medication you have on hand and how much you will need while on vacation. If it looks as if you may run out of medications before returning home, have your doctor call in refills that you can pick up before you leave. If your insurance company says it is too soon for refills, talk with your doctor; he or she can request an exception, explaining to the insurance company that you will be away from home when it will be time for refills. If possible, keep an extra supply of medications with you in case you are away from home longer than expected.

Keep Your Pharmacy Information with You — Make certain you carry your pharmacy information with you while traveling. It is a good idea to have the pharmacy name, telephone number, and fax number in your purse or wallet. That way, if you run out of medications while away from home, a pharmacy near where you are vacationing can contact your local pharmacy to transfer prescription information, allowing you to get a refill while you're away. It's also a good idea to find a pharmacy near where you'll be staying while away from home. If you use a large pharmacy chain, find an outlet near your vacation spot. That will make transferring prescriptions much easier in the event you will need to fill your prescriptions away from home.

Known Your Physician's Office Number / Have Your Insurance Information — Make certain you carry your doctor's name, office number, and fax number with you while away from home. Keep a copy of this information in your wallet or purse, and another copy with your luggage. In the event you or a pharmacy needs to call for new prescriptions, having the information on hand will make getting refills much easier. Have your insurance information on hand as well in order to pay for any prescriptions you get refilled while away from home.

Keep Your Medications with You — If you are traveling by air, train, or bus, make certain you have your medications in your carry-on luggage, not in the bags you have checked and stowed in the luggage compartment. First, having them in your carry-on luggage allows access to them if you need to take a dose while en route to your destination. Second, your checked baggage can be lost or tampered with, meaning your medications could be lost as well. Keep in mind that security measures on airplanes limit the amount of liquid you can carry on your person to about three ounces. Check with your airline well in advance of your departure date to get specific rules and limitations regarding liquid medication rules. If your dose and type of medication allows, switch to tablet or capsule form while travelling, and then switch back to liquid if you prefer upon your return.

Store Your Medication Properly — When at all possible, keep your prescription medications in the bottle you received from the pharmacy. Make sure you keep the bottle's label in place as well. The prescription information contained on the label will help you prove the medications you are carrying are your prescriptions. Taking medications out of prescription bottles will delay your time through security. Certain HIV medications — specifically, soft gel capsules— require special handling and storage. If they get too warm, they will melt and stick together. Do not leave them in your car, near a heat source, in the sunlight, or anywhere else where they can get too warm. Ideally they should be refrigerated, so request a hotel room with a small refrigerator if available. If the hotel does not have refrigerators in the room, bring a small cooler or use the room's ice bucket to keep them cool. Place the prescription bottle in a plastic bag and place the plastic bag on ice, keeping the medication cool but not so cold that it freezes.

Needles and Syringes —If you have been prescribed injectable medication, the medication and syringes must be carried together in order to be allowed in your carry-on. Do not take the syringes out of their sterile packaging; syringes not in packaging may be confiscated or at the very least will slow your time through security. Once again, make certain you keep labels on all injectable prescription medication to make it easier for security to identify the medications as belonging to you.

You Are Entitled to Privacy —If airport security feels they need to question you regarding your medications, or for any reason during the screening process, you are entitled to privacy and confidentiality. It is within your rights to request that the questioning be done in a private area.

Special Travel Considerations

Traveling with an HIV diagnosis presents problems that few others experience. We discussed special measures that can make travel with medications less problematic, but there are other issues outside of those surrounding your HIV regimen. There are special considerations that must be taken into account in order to travel safely when living with an HIV diagnosis. Depending on your destination, there can be health concerns associated with your travel. Water-borne illnesses, infectious diseases, or other epidemics can present a risk to anyone with a weakened immune system, HIV-positive people included. But there are steps that can be taken to minimize the risk.

Before You Travel

- Speak with your doctor about any possible health risks associated with your destination. For instance, are you traveling to a part of the world where you may be at increased risk for hepatitis A? Is malaria a problem where you are vacationing? Is the water safe to drink? Large hospitals or university clinics typically have travel clinics that specialize in preparing you for travel to places outside the U.S. Depending on your destination, you may require certain vaccinations to protect you from illnesses common to the area you're visiting. To make certain your body has time to respond to any vaccinations you may require, visit a travel clinic a few months before your departure.
- Depending on the area you are heading to, *"traveler's diarrhea"* may be a

problem. Traveler's diarrhea is a condition that results from ingesting food or water contaminated with diarrhea-causing microbes. Usually it's an affliction that occurs when you travel from areas of good sanitation to poor. Your doctor can prescribe an antibiotic you can fill and carry with you to start taking at the first sign of diarrhea.

- Insect-borne illnesses such as malaria may be present at your destination. Take plenty of insect repellent with you when traveling. Also, make sure you sleep under mosquito netting in those areas where mosquitoes are known to carry diseases that may put you at risk for illness.
- If you are leaving the United States, check with the countries you are visiting before your trip to see if that country has any special health requirements or rules pertaining to HIV. Be aware that some countries require vaccinations that are unsafe for people with HIV (e.g., live vaccines). If that is the case, you will need a letter from your doctor explaining why you are unable to take that particular vaccine.
- Check with your medical insurance to learn the extent of coverage if you are traveling out of the country or out of the network area. Take proof of insurance with you, regardless of where you travel.

While Away from Home

- If you are traveling out of the United States, be aware that the quality of water may not be what you are accustomed to. In fact, it may be very poor. In some cases there are parasites and bacteria in the water that makes it unsafe to drink. In these areas drink only commercially bottled water. Rinse your toothbrush and your mouth with the same bottled water to avoid exposure to parasites or bacteria that may be in the local drinking water. The same precautions are advised if you are camping in the wild and get your water from streams or ponds. Do not eat raw fruit or vegetables you have not cleaned and peeled yourself. Do not drink local tap water; do not drink any mixed drinks made with tap water; and do not use ice made from tap water.
- Avoid any foods from local street vendors. Eat only those foods deemed safe, including those that are steaming hot, those you have cleaned and peeled yourself, and water that you have brought to a rolling boil for at least a full minute.
- Tuberculosis (TB) is a common disease outside of the United States. If you must go to a hospital or clinic while you are traveling, avoid people with productive coughs, fevers, or other signs of respiratory illness. Use only clinics or medical facilities that are clean and use sterile equipment.
- In many parts of the world, domesticated farm animals such as cows and chickens are left to roam free. Do not swim in any water or walk any beach you suspect may be contaminated with animal droppings or waste. Never

drink or swallow water while you are swimming, and avoid opening your eyes under the water.

HIV Prevention, Diagnosis and Beyond

Our journey from HIV prevention to diagnosis and beyond has come to a close. It's my wish that this text will help you cope with your illness, help you understand your disease, and finally help you live with HIV. This text is complete, but your journey with HIV continues. If I could give you one piece of advice, I would say learn everything you can about your disease. Knowledge is power, so learn all you can and take control of your disease; in doing so you will take control of your life.

Live healthy...

Bibliography

AIDS 101: Guide to HIV Basics. San Francisco AIDS Foundation, 1998.

Altman, L.K. "Rare Cancer Seen in 41 Homosexuals." *The New York Times*, July 3, 1981.

"Americans Awaken to the AIDS Crisis, 1985." *The Wall Street Journal*, December 12, 1989, p. B1.

Ammann, A. "Counseling HIV-Infected Patients Who Want to Have Children." March 2006 [cited 2008 March 3]. Available from: http://www.womenchildrenhiv.org/wchiv?page=tp-02-01.

Anderson, R.N., and B.L Smith. "Deaths: Leading Causes for 2002." *National Vital Statistics Report*, 2005, 53(17).

Anil, S.N., R.G. Nair, V.T. Beena, and T. Vijuyakumar. "Dental Professionals' Attitude and Knowledge Towards HIV Infection and AIDS — An Indian Perspective." *Community Dentistry and Oral Epidemiology*, 1995, 23(3), pp. 187–188.

Arquin, P.M., P.E. Kozarsky, and C. Reed, eds. *CDC Health Information for International Travel 2008.* Chapter 4: "Prevention of Infectious Diseases— Travelers Diarrhea." Atlanta: Centers for Disease Control, 2008, p. 648.

Atif, M.S. "Low CD4+ Nadir Is an Independent Predictor of Lower HIV-Specific Immune Responses in Chronically HIV-1 Infected Subjects Receiving Highly Active Antiretroviral Therapy." *The Journal of Infectious Disease*, 2006, 194, pp. 661–665.

Barry, A.M., J.G. Kahn, S.D. Pinkerton, et al. "Postexposure Prophylaxis Following HIV Exposure." *Journal of the American Medical Association*, 1999, 281(14), p. 1269.

Bartlett, J.G., and R.D. Moore. "Improving HIV Therapy." *Scientific American*, 1998, 279(1), pp. 84–87, 89.

Biel-Cunningham, S. "The Importance of Dental Care." *Survival News*, November/December 2004.

Bryg, R. "High Cholesterol: Cholesterol Basics," *Cholesterol Management Guide.* Cleveland: Cleveland Clinic Foundation, 2006.

Buchaman, M.J.W, and L. Kent. "What Makes Cryptococcus a Pathogen?" *Emerging Infectious Diseases*, 1998, 4(1), pp. 71–83.

Carter, N. "Support Groups: Places of Healing." *HIV/AIDS*, 1994 (Focus Paper #23).

Castro, K.G. "1993 Revised Classification System for HIV Infection and Expanded Surveillance Case Definition for AIDS Among Adolescents and Adults." *CDC Mortality and Morbidity Weekly Report*, 1992, 44 (No. RR-17).

Cichocki, M.W. "Bacterial Opportunistic Infections," *HIV/AIDS* at About.com 2004 1/2004 [cited 2007 August 3]. Available from: http://aids.about.com/cs/conditions/a/bacterialoi.htm.

_____. "How to Choose the Right HIV Doctor," 2005 [cited 2005 3/10/05]. Available from: http://www.suite101.com/article.cfm/hivaids/114901.

_____. "Side Effects, Symptoms, and Solutions," *HIV/AIDS* at About.com 2003 8/1/03 [cited 2007 February 4]. Available from: http://aids.about.com/cs/conditions/a/sides.htm.

Cornforth, T. "Abnormal Pap Smears." *Women's Health* at About.com 2003 12/7/03 [cited 2007 November 18]. Available from: http://womenshealth.about.com/cs/pap smears/a/abnormalpaps.htm.

_____. "Understanding Your Pap Smear Results," *Women's Health* at About.com 2007 9/1/07 [cited 2008 April 3]; Available from: http://womenshealth.about.com/cs/papsmears/a/papsmearresults.htm.

Davenport, T. "How to Prevent Gum Disease." Dental Care at About.com 2007 3/28/07 [cited 2007 December 19]. Available from: http://dentistry.about.com/od/tooth mouthconditions/ht/preventing.htm.

Drainoni, M.L. *Reports and Studies: Substance Abuse and HIV*. H.A. Bureau, ed. Health Resources Services Administration (HRSA), 2003.

Eversole, L.R, A.S. Leider, P.L. Jacobson, and E.P. Shaber. "Oral Kaposi's Sarcoma Associated with Acquired Immunodeficiency Syndrome Among Homosexual Males." *Journal of American Dentistry Association*, 1983, 107(2), pp. 248–253.

Fact Sheet Number 802: Exercise and HIV. New Mexico AIDS Infonet Fact Sheets 2008 4/14/08 [cited 2008 January 18].

Ferri, J. *There Is Hope: Learning to Live with HIV*. 2d ed. HIV Coalition, 1998.

Fischbach, F. *A Manual of Laboratory and Diagnostic Tests*. 7th. ed. Philadelphia: Lippincott, Williams and Wilkins, 2004.

Fox, M. *Study: AIDS Prevention Saved Up to 1.5 Million*. November 26, 2002. Available from: http://www.thebody.com/content/treat/art18742.html.

Fudala, P.J., et al. "Office Base Treatment of Opiate Addiction with a Sublingual Tablet Formulation of Buprenorphine and Naloxone." *New England Journal of Medicine*, 2003, 349(10), pp. 949–958.

Functional Foods Fact Sheet: Antioxidants. Fact Sheets 2006, March 2006. Available from: http://www.ific.org/publications/factsheets/antioxidantfs.cfm.

Gottlieb, M. "Pneumocystis Pneumonia in Los Angeles." *CDC Mortality and Morbidity Weekly Report*, 1981(30), pp. 250–252.

Grodeck, B. *The First Year — HIV: An Essential Guide for the Newly Diagnosed*. 2d ed. New York: Perseus, 2007.

Hader, S.L, D.K. Smith, J.S. Moore, and S. D. Holmberg. "HIV Infection in Women in the United States." *Journal of the American Medical Association*, 2001, 285(9), pp. 1186–1192.

Hilton, B. "AIDS Week — Reagan: Better Late Than Never?" *San Francisco Sunday Examiner and Chronicle*, 1990, San Francisco, p. A4.

Hinman, A. "Researchers Trace First HIV Case to 1959 in the Belgian Congo." 1998 2/3/1998 [cited 2006 August 8]. Available from: http://www.cnn.com/HEALTH/9802/03/earliest.aids/.

"HIV Treatment Education: Community Perspectives." *ACRIA Update*, 2002, 11(4), pp. 1–20.

"HIV Treatment Information: Lipodystrophy Syndrome(s)." 2001 11/1/01; Available from: http://www.projinf.org/fs/lipo.html.

The HIV/AIDS Program: Ryan White Parts A-F. 2008 [cited 2007 March 5]. Available from: http://hab.hrsa.gov/aboutus.htm.

Horsburgh, R. "Antiretroviral Therapy Reduces Risk of Bacterial Pneumonia." *American Journal of Respiratory Critical Care Medicine*, July 2000.

Johanson, D. *A Practical Guide to Nutrition for People Living with HIV*. 2d ed. Canadian AIDS Treatment Information Exchange (CATIE), 2007.

Kennedy, I., and S. Williams. "Occupational Exposure to HIV and Post-Exposure

Prophylaxis in Healthcare Workers." *Occupational Medicine*, 2000, 50(6), pp. 387–391.

Krist, A.H., and A. Crawford-Faucher. "Management of Newborns Exposed to Maternal HIV Infection." *American Family Physician*, 2002, 65(10), pp. 2049–2058.

Krist, M.D., and H. Alex. "Obstetrics Care in Patients with HIV Disease." *American Family Physician*, 2001.

Kusmer, K. "Farewell to the Young Symbol of Courage." *Washington Post*, date unknown 1990, p. C1.

Lab Tests Online. 2001–2005 [cited 5/3/08]. Available from: http://www.labtestsonline. org/understanding/analytes/viral_load/test.html.

Lawson-Ayayi, S. "Avascular Necrosis in HIV-Infected Patients: A Case-Control Study from the Aquitane Cohort, 1997–2002 France." *Clinical Infectious Disease*, 2005, 40(8), pp. 1188–1193.

Lee, D. "Canker Sores (Apthous Ulcers)." 2005, 10/6/05 [cited 2007 November 7]. Available from: http://www.medicinenet.com/canker_sores/article.htm.

Linnemeyer, P.A. "*The Immune System — An Overview.*" November 1993 [cited 10/11/08]. Available from: http://www.thebody.com/content/art1788.html.

Lipodystrophy. June 2002 [cited Fact Sheet 39]. Available from: http://www.aidsmap. com/en/docs/pdf/fs39.pdf.

Marsh, L.A. "Comparison of Pharmacological Treatment for Opioid Dependent Adolescents: A Randomized Control Trial." *Archives of General Psychiatry*, 2005, 62(10), pp. 1157–1164.

McEwan, M. *Pneumocystis Jiroveci Pneumonia*, 2008, 9/30/08. Available from: http://en. wikipedia.org/wiki/Pneumocystis_pneumonia.

Mirken, B. "HIV Testing 101." *AIDS Treatment News*, 2001, p. 374.

"The Most Common Opportunistic Infections in Women with HIV." *HIV Newsline*, 1998 [cited 2008 April 5]. Available from: http://www.thebody.com/content/art 12622.html.

National Treatment Improvement Evaluation Study (NTIES): Highlights. U.S. Department of Health and Human Services, Substance Abuse and Mental Health Services Administration. 1997, pp. 241–242.

Nauert, R. "Why Mental Illness and Addiction Occur Together." *Psych Central News*, 2007 [cited 2007 December 3]. Available from: http://psychcentral.com/news/ 2007/12/03/why-mental-illness-and-addiction-occur-together/1602.html.

Nerad, J., M. Romeyn, E. Silverman, et al. "General Nutrition Management in Patients Infected with Human Immunodeficiency Virus." *Clinical Infectious Disease*, 2003, 36(Supplement 2), pp. 552–562.

Padiun, N. "*HIV and Heterosexual Gender Gap — Man to Woman Transmission More Likely Than Woman to Man.*" 1991, 10/5/91 [cited 2008 July 28]. Available from: http://findarticles.com/p/articles/mi_m1200/is_n14_v140/ai_11489577.

Palmer, M. *Dr. Melissa Palmer's Guide to Hepatitis and Liver Disease: What You Need to Know*. New York: Penquin Putnam, 2004.

Pedezanin, S. "Fear of Dentists." 2002 [cited 2008 May 17]. Available from: http://www. essortment.com/all/feardentists_rcos.htm.

Penn, M. *Fighting Heart Disease: Should You Be "Pro" or "Anti" Antioxidants?* Cleveland Clinic Heart and Vascular Institute, 2008.

Powderly, W.G. "Effect of Opportunistic Illness on Risk of Death in HIV Disease." *Journal of the American Medical Association*, 1998, 279(18), p. 1500.

"Psychosocial Support HIV/AIDS." November 2007. Available from: http://www.who. int/hiv/topics/psychosocial/support/en.

Quan, K. "Issues Affecting Patient Education." 2004. Available from: http://nursing. about.com/od/patienteducation/a/patienteduc.html.

Rabkin, J. "The Good HIV Patient." In *Good Patients, Good Doctors*. New York: NCM, 1994.

Randall, M.C. "Support Groups: What They Are and What They Do." *Genetic Health*, December 2003.

Recer, P. "Education Helps Patient Health." *Associated Press*, 2002.

"Recommendations for Prevention and Control of Hepatitis C Virus (HCV) Infection and HCV Related Chronic Disease." *Morbidity and Mortality Weekly Report*, 1998, 47(No. RR-19), pp. 1–54.

Reichart, P. "Oral Manifestations in HIV: Fungal and Bacterial Infections; Kaposi's Sarcoma." *Medical Microbiology and Immunology*, 2003, 192(3), pp. 165–169.

Reiter, G. "The HIV Wasting Syndrome," *AIDS Clinical Care*, 1996.

Reznik, D. *"Perspective: Oral Manifestations of HIV Disease,"* in *8th Annual Clinical Conference for the Ryan White CARE Act Clinicians*, New Orleans, LA, 2005.

_____. "Recognition and Management of the Most Common Oral Manifestations of HIV Infection." 1999 [cited 2008 January 19]. Available from: http://www.thebody.com/content/treat/art2806.html.

Sanders, A. "HIV-Associated Bacterial Pneumonia." *The AIDS Reader*, 1999, 9(8), pp. 580–583.

Scott, J. "What Is a Calorie and Why Should I Care?" 2008, 3/17/08 [cited 2008 May 18]. Available from: http://weightloss.about.com/od/nutrition/a/blwhatcal.htm.

Siegal, H.A., R.S. Falck, R.G. Carlson, and J. Wang. "Reducing HIV Needle Risk Behaviors Among Injection-Drug Users in the Midwest: An Evaluation of the Efficacy of Stand and Enhanced Interventions." *AIDS Education and Prevention*, 1995, 7(4), pp. 308–319.

Sikkema, K. "Predictors of AIDS-Related Grief Among HIV-Infected Men and Women." In *International Conference on AIDS*. Durban, South Africa, 2000.

Slanetz, L.W., and E.A. Brown. "Studies on the Number of Bacteria in the Mouth and Their Reduction by the Use of Oral Antiseptics." *Journal of Dental Research*, 1949, 23(3), pp. 313–323.

Speakes, L. "White House Press Briefing." 1982, Office of the Press Secretary, Washington, D.C.

Sreebny, L., and S.S. Schwartz. "Treatment of Drug-Induced Xerostomia." 2008 [cited 2008 May 16]; Available from: http://www.drymouth.info/practitioner/treatment.asp.

Stafford, N.D. "Kaposi's Sarcoma of the Head and Neck in Patients with AIDS." *The Journal of Laryngology and Otology*, 1989(103), pp. 379–382.

"Starting HIV Treatment — New Guidelines and Questions." The Simple Facts Project 2008 4/12/08 [cited 5/19/08]. Available from: http://www.atdn.org/simple/guidelines.html.

Timpe, J.M., et al. "Hepatitis C Virus Cell-Cell Transmission Hepatoma Cells in the Presence of Neutralizing Antibodies." *Hepatology*, 2007(47), pp. 17–24.

Tofferi, J.K. "Avascular Necrosis." *Emedicine*, January 2006. Available from: http://emedicine.medscape.com/article/333364-overview.

Tsang, G. "Fiber 101: Soluble Fiber vs. Insoluble Fiber." 2005 [cited 11/2005]. Available from: http://www.healthcastle.com/fiber-solubleinsoluble.shtml.

Understanding the Immune System — How It Works. U.S. Department of Health and Human Services. National Institute of Allergy and Infectious Diseases, National Institutes of Health and National Cancer Institute, 2003.

Vernazza, P., et al. "HIV-Discordant Couples and Parenthood: How Are They Dealing with the Risk of Transmission." *AIDS*, 2006, 20(4), pp. 635–636.

Volkow, N. "What Do We Know About Addiction?" *American Journal of Psychology*, 2005(162), pp. 1401–1402.

Von Roenn, J. "Treatment of HIV-Associated Kaposi's Sarcoma." *HIV Insite's Knowledge Base,* June 2003 [cited 2007 April 4]. Available from: http://hivinsite.ucsf.edu/InSite?page=kb-06-02-04.

Waknine, Y. "Highlights from MMWR: Decline in Adult Smoking Stalls and More." *Morbidity and Mortality Weekly Report,* 2006(55), pp. 1145–1168.

Watson, J. "Five Lessons on Motivation from a Visit to the Dentist." 2008 [cited 2008 May 18]. Available from: http://ezinearticles.com/?Five-Lessons-On-Motivation-From-A-Visit-To-The-Dentist&id=116094.

"Why Should I Be Tested — The Benefits of Knowing." AIDS.org 2005. Available from: http://www.sfaf.org/aids101/hiv_testing.html.

Woolston, C. "Finding a Dentist." 2003, 2/11/08 [cited 2003 March 4]. Available from: http://www.yourhealthconnection.com/topic/dentist.

Workowski, K., and S.M. Berman. *"Mortality and Morbidity Weekly Report — Sexually Transmitted Diseases Treatment Guidelines, 2006."* National Center for HIV/AIDS, Viral Hepatitis, STD, and TB Prevention, 2006.

Zickler, P. *Buprenorphine Plus Behavioral Therapy Is Effective for Adolescents with Opioid Addiction.* National Institute on Drug Abuse (NIDA), 2006.

Zorilla, C.D. "Women Living with HIV: An Evolving Story." In *11t. Annual Clinical Update.* Washington, D.C.: The International AIDS Society, 2008.

Index